Immunit

How Anima

DATE DUE			

To the Memory of G.J.W.

There is nothing funny in the thought that even man, who was made in the image of God, bears about in his vital organs various forms of loathsome creatures, which riot on his fluids and consume the very substance of his tissues.

Philip Henry Gosse

Immunity to Parasites

How Animals Control Parasitic Infections

Derek Wakelin
Ph.D., D.Sc.
Professor of Zoology, University of Nottingham

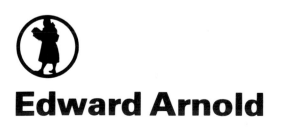

Edward Arnold

First published in Great Britain 1984
by Edward Arnold (Publishers) Ltd,
41 Bedford Square,
London WC1B 3DQ

Edward Arnold (Australia) Pty Ltd,
80 Waverley Road,
Caulfield East,
Victoria 3145,
Australia

Edward Arnold,
300 North Charles Street,
Baltimore,
Maryland 212001,
U.S.A.

ISBN 0 7131 2889 5

Text set in 9/10 Times
by The Castlefield Press
Printed and bound in Great Britain by
Thomson Litho Ltd, East Kilbride, Scotland

Preface

Parasitic animals constitute one of the major causes of the infectious diseases which affect man and his domestic animals. The cumulative effects of parasitism in terms of mortality, chronic disease and economic loss are incalculably great and undoubtedly play an important part in limiting the social and economic development of many countries in sub-tropical and tropical regions of the world. It should not be thought that man and domestic stock are in some way uniquely vulnerable to parasitic infections. All species are subject to infection by a characteristic assemblage of parasitic animals adapted to them, and these relationships have arisen as a result of long evolutionary development. Exploitation of the environments provided by the bodies of living animals is, in essence, no different from the exploitation of the environments provided by the seas, the land and fresh waters, and has been a major line of evolution followed by species from many phyla. The success of this way of life is reflected in the extent to which animals of every phylum are parasitized and in the stability and antiquity of many host–parasite relationships. Stability is often reflected in minimal incovenience to the life and survival of the host and is dependent upon a balanced relationship not only between individual hosts and individual parasites, but also between populations of each. Thus, although man and domestic stock are not exceptional in their susceptibility to parasites, both may live under conditions which predispose them to heavy and continuous infection. In consequence the balance of the host–parasite relationship is disturbed and the host may suffer severely from parasite disease.

The almost universal occurrence of parasites has exerted a major influence upon the evolution of the protective responses which allow hosts to regulate the levels of infections to which they are subject. All hosts have the capacity to respond adaptively to the presence of parasites and to exert deleterious effects upon their growth and survival. All parasites, therefore, have had to evolve strategies by which they can circumvent these effects. In higher vertebrates this adaptive response is very largely, though not exclusively, the property of the immune system, and immunologically-based, anti-parasite responses represent a major survival strategy. The study of these responses has obvious relevance to human and veterinary medicine, particularly in the search for more effective means of control, and in recent years has attracted a great deal of research interest from both parasitologists and immunologists. Warren has differentiated between 'parasite-immunologists', trained in immunology, and 'immuno-parasitologists', trained in parasitology. Both, however, are required to make biologically meaningful studies of immune responses to parasites. Each complements the other, and the growth of their research field, which I prefer to call immunoparasitology, is a satisfying example of mutualism in action.

Immunoparasitology has an obvious applied significance. It is also an intriguing area of study in its own right, throwing light upon fundamental aspects of protective immune responses and illuminating the intricacies of host-parasite interactions. The results of immunoparasitological research are now published in a wide variety of journals and have been summarized in a number of excellent texts and reviews. Few of these sources are entirely appropriate for the undergraduate or graduate biologist seeking an insight into the immunological aspects of parasitology, or for the immunologist wishing to put immunoparasitology into an biological context. The aim of this volume is to meet these needs by concentrating on selected host–parasite relationships in which immunologically-orientated research has made significant progress, both in elucidating the nature of host-protective responses and in clarifying the reciprocal interactions between these responses and parasite adaptations. The introductory chapters are intended to help readers of differing backgrounds into the subject area. That on immunology is designed primarily to introduce aspects of the immune response which are relevant to immunoparasitology. Chapters 4 to 9 then consider a limited number of examples chosen to illustrate the diversity of organisms and adaptations with which the immune response must deal. The emphasis in these chapters falls upon experimental studies using laboratory model systems, in which particular problems can be analysed in great detail without the many complicating factors that bedevil analysis of protective responses in man and domestic animals. Nevertheless, the ultimate goal of experimental studies is to provde data applicable to the understanding and the control of human and animal disease, and the final chapter considers the ways in which such studies are contributing to this objective.

This is not intended to be a comprehensive account of immunoparasitology and, inevitably, much that can rightly be considered significant has had to be omitted. It is very much a personal overview; nevertheless, it will, I hope, be useful to a wide variety of readers and contribute a little to the growth and development of a fascinating science.

Nottingham, 1984   D.W.

Acknowledgements

I am very grateful to my colleagues in the Department of Zoology at Nottingham for their advice and helpful suggestions on the content and presentation of this book. Mr W.J. Haddow gave valuable assistance with preparation of some of the plates. My thanks go to Miss W. Lister and Mrs C.A. Taylor for their patience and accuracy in producing the typed manuscript.

All drawings which are not original have been adpated from the sources acknowledged in the legends. I am greatly indebted to the following individuals, publishers and copyright holders for their permission to reproduce their photographs:
Plate 4.1, Dr R.S. Nussenzweig and Academic Press; Plate 4.2, Dr R.S. Nussenzweig and *Journal of Immunology* (American Association of Immunologists); Plate 4.3, Dr L.H. Bannister and *Parasitology* (Cambridge University Press); Plate 4.4, Dr R.E. Sinden; Plates 4.5 (a), Dr J. Alexander and Academic Press; Plate 4.5 (b), Dr J. Alexander and *Transactions of the Royal Society for Tropical Medicine and Hygiene*; Plates 5.1 and 5.2, Mr L. Tetley and Professor K. Vickerman; Plates 6.1 and 6.2 (a), Dr A.M. Glauert and Dr A.E. Butterworth; Plates 6.2 (b) and (d), Dr D.J. McLaren and *Parasitology* (Cambridge University Press); Plate 6.2 (c), Dr D.J. McLaren and Research Studies Press; Plate 7.1; Dr K.A. Wright and *Journal of Parasitology* (American Society of Parasitology); Plate 7.2, Dr H. Alizadeh; Plate 8.1, Dr N.W.T. Clarke, Dr R.M.E. Parkhouse and *Biochemical Journal* (Biochemical Society); Plate 8.2, Dr D.J. McLaren; Plate 8.3, Dr A. Haque and *Journal of Immunology* (American Association of Immunologists); Plate 9.1, Dr S.J. Brown; Plate 9.2, Dr S.J. Brown and *Experimental Parasitology* (Academic Press).

Contents

1

Parasites and Parasitism

The Host as an Environment

In many older textbooks of Zoology it was customary to treat parasite species as though they were in some way quite separate from free-living animals. The term 'degenerate', which was used to describe the apparent simplifications in structure shown by parasites when compared with their free-living relatives, also carried with it a whiff of moral disapproval for their way of life! Today the pendulum has swung almost to the other extreme and parasitism is sometimes represented as nothing more than another form of environmental exploitation. It is indeed a remarkably successful exploitation and one that has been a major line of evolutionary development in several phyla. The success of this way of life is attested by the ubiquity of parasites, in hosts of every phylum, and in the long-term stability of many host–parasite relationships. In essence, of course, it is true that exploitation of the host environment is very similar to the exploitation of any other environment, but there is one very important difference. Unlike the environments of free-living animals, the environment provided by a host can respond adaptively to the presence of a parasite. It is this difference, the adaptive interaction of host and parasite, each concerned with its own evolutionary survival, that distinguishes parasitism from other modes of life.

1.1   What is a Parasite?

Despite the distinctive feature outlined above it is almost impossible to define parasitism in terms which completely exclude related modes of interspecific association such as commensalism and mutualism. In the host–parasite relationship the parasite is undoubtedly the beneficiary, but the precise requirements for parasite survival and the extent to which the host may suffer from the association are extremely variable. For the purposes of this book, which will be concerned almost exclusively with endoparasites in warm-blooded hosts (Table 1.1), it is useful to apply some ecological concepts in describing the essential characteristics of the parasitic way of life.

For parasites the host is the total environment. Larval and other reproductive stages may live in the outside world for longer or shorter periods but this represents merely a necessary phase in the movement from host to host. Particular parasites occupy particular niches in the major habitats provided by the host environment and are adapted to the conditions present in those niches in exactly the same way as free-living organisms are adapted to their environments. Although the environment

Table 1.1 Table of major parasites referred to in the text.

Classification	Genus	Position in host	Transmission	Size
Protozoa				
Mastigophora	*Trypanosoma*	Extracellular/Blood	Bite of tsetse fly	15–25 μm
	Leishmania	Intracellular/Macrophage	Bite of sandfly	2–5 μm
Apicomplexa	*Plasmodium*	Intracellular/RBC	Bite of mosquito	2–20 μm
Platyhelminthes				
Digenea	*Schistosoma*	Blood vessels (adults)	Skin penetration by larvae	10–30 mm ($\female$)
Nematoda				
Strongylida	Hookworms, *Haemonchus*, *Nippostrongylus*, *Trichostrongylus*, *Nematospiroides*	Intestinal lumen	Oral ingestion or skin penetration by larvae	$\simeq 10$ mm ($\female$)
	Dictyocaulus	Lungs		10 cm ($\female$)
Trichinelloidea	*Trichinella*	Intracellular/Gut epithelium	Oral ingestion of larvae	2–3 mm ($\female$)
Filaroidea	*Wuchereria*, *Brugia*	Lymphatics (adults)	Bite of mosquito	100 mm ($\female$)
	Onchocerca	Subcutaneous tissue (adults)	Bite of *Simulium*	500 mm ($\female$)
Arthropoda				
Acarina	"Ticks"	Ectoparasitic on skin	Direct host contact	5–15 mm ($\female$)

is wholly biotic in origin, as it is provided by a living organism, it is still possible to define each niche by what are essentially abiotic factors such as pH, oxygen tension, redox potential and nutrient availability, as well as truly biotic factors such as other parasites and resident microorganisms. The ecological analogies break down, however, when one considers that the environment provided by the host is not passive, but can react adaptively to the presence of the parasite. Thus even in an environment to which they are perfectly adapted, parasites are faced by a variety of potentially destructive factors never experienced by free-living species, for example antibodies, complement components, cytotoxins, lysosmal enzymes, as well as predatory phagocytic cells. The ability of the parasite to evade or resist these adaptive responses ultimately determines the ability of the parasite to survive and reproduce.

An important consequence of the endoparasitic condition is that the parasite is cut off from direct experience of the external world. Some parasites still rely on external changes in temperature and daylength, which they perceive indirectly through the hormonal and other changes in the host, to control their own developmental processes. Other (e.g. intestinal nematodes of sheep) use their direct experience of these changes, whilst they are in the external world as larval stages, to regulate their development after entry into the host. Nevertheless, the majority coordinate their growth, development and reproduction by responding to factors present within the host environment which have little or no relationship to the outside world. Such adaptations have clear selective advantage in preventing developmental changes from taking place in the absence of suitable hosts.

1.2 Parasite Life Cycles

There is an almost infinite variety of ways in which parasites reach their hosts and of life cycles directed to this end, but it is possible to reduce this variety to a number of basic patterns.

1. The parasite is never exposed to the external world and completes its development and reproduction in a single host. Relatively few parasites show this pattern. Transmission between hosts is normally achieved by carnivory (Fig. 1.1a).
2. The parasite is never exposed to the external world, but its developmental cycle takes place in two or more host species. The species in which the parasite reaches sexual maturity is known as the *final* or *definitive* host; that in which larval, juvenile or non-sexual stages develop is known as the *intermediate* host. Where one host transmits the parasite directly to another it is also referred to as a vector and this term is applied particularly to arthropods (Fig. 1.1b).
3. The parasite is exposed to the external world for varying periods of time, but does not have active, free-living stages. The infective forms are contained within protective structures such as cysts (Protozoa) or egg shells (Nematoda). The life cycle may be *direct* in that only one host species is involved, or *indirect*, involving intermediate and final hosts of different species (Figs 1.1c and 1.1d).
4. The parasite is exposed to the external world as an active, free-living form during its development and transmission between hosts. Re-entry into the host may be a passive process, i.e. by ingestion, or an active process by penetration. As before the cycle may be direct or indirect (Figs 1.1e and 1.1f).

In all patterns, certain phases in the life cycle act as the infective stages and these may show well-defined morphological or physiological adaptations for this function. These are particularly evident in the skin-penetrating larvae of helminths, for example the cercariae of schistosomes, which possess suckers for adhesion and a battery of glandular structures which release histolytic enzymes. Characteristic of all

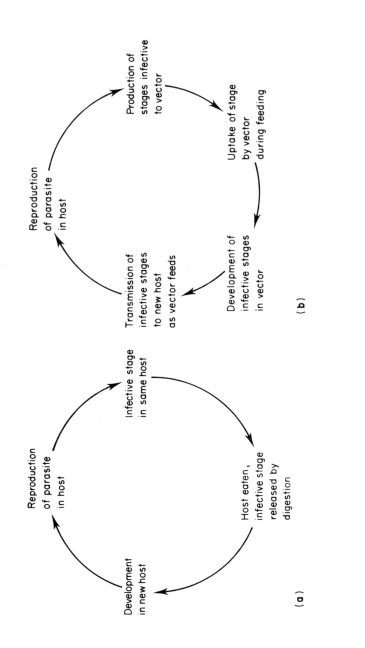

Fig. 1.1 Life Cycles of Endoparasites.
(a) Direct cycle, parasite never exposed to the outside world, transmission by carnivory, e.g. *Trichinella spiralis* (Nematoda).
(b) Indirect cycle, parasite never exposed to the outside world, transmission by arthropod vector, e.g. *Plasmodium* (Protozoa), *Wuchereria* (Nematoda).

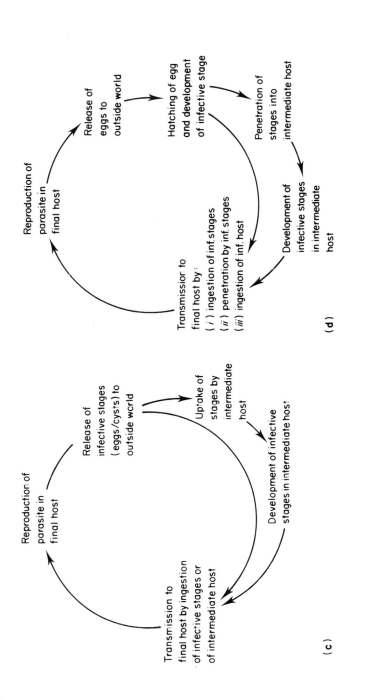

Fig. 1.1 *cont.*
(**c**) Direct and indirect cycles, parasite exposed to the outside world but not as an active free-living stage. Transmission direct, e.g. *Toxoplasma* (Protozoa), *Ascaris* (Nematoda), or indirect via an intermediate host, e.g. tapeworms (Platyhelminthes).
(**d**) Direct and indirect cycles, parasite exposed to the outside world as free-living stage. Transmission direct, e.g. hookworms, *Haemonchus* (Nematoda), or indirect via an intermediate host, e.g. *Schistosoma* (Platyhelminthes).

infective stages is the capacity to recognize the host environment. In protozoan infective stages such as the malarial sporozoite, this capacity operates at a molecular level and involves complementarity between surface receptors of host cells and molecules present on the parasite. In the infective stages of helminths, particularly those which enter the host in a protective sheath, cyst or eggshell, recognition of the host involves response to certain physico-chemical stimuli that act as triggers to initiate escape from the protective layers and recommencement of growth and development. Clearly, despite numerous adaptations to ensure that it is the correct host species which is invaded, there is a large random element in the process. Host contact may or may not be made. If made, infection may fail because the host is unsuitable. The reasons underlying failures of the latter kind can be very instructive because, by throwing light upon the phenomenon of natural resistance or natural insusceptibility to infection, they reveal much about the characteristics of the susceptible host.

1.3   Natural Resistance to Infection

Natural resistance is a phenomenon operating at many levels (Table 1.2). Hosts can be considered naturally resistant to parasites because, through geographical distribution, behavioural characteristics or nutritional habits, they simply do not come into contact with infective stages. (Man's natural resistance to many parasites is clearly of this kind and all too frequently breaks down.) Natural resistance more

Table 1.2   Influence of factors involved in natural resistance and acquired resistance to parasitic infection. Natural resistance is expressed through the host's behaviour, structure and physiology; acquired resistance is expressed through the host's immune response. The two categories are not absolute, each is intimately related to the other.

Stage in host parasite infection	*Host characteristics which influence Interaction*			
	Behaviour	Structure	Physiology	Immunity
Initial contact	+	+	−	−
Establishment in host	−	+	+	−
Development of parasite	−	+	+	+
Reproduction of parasite	−	−	+	+

conventionally encompasses a physiological incompatibility between parasite and host environment which prevents invasion, establishment or survival without the intervention of immunologically-based protective responses.

Incompatibility may be evident during the initial stage of infection. For example:

(a) Helminths, such as schistosomes and hookworms that rely on skin-penetrating larvae for infection may be unable to successfully cross the epidermis and basement membrane in order to enter the dermis.

(b) Trypanosomes entering the blood may be killed by factors naturally present in serum, such as the high density lipo-protein which destroys animal-infective *T.b. brucei* in man, or may activate complement and be lysed.

(c) Intracellular protozoa such as *Plasmodium* may be unable to enter host cells because essential surface receptors are absent.

(*d*) Parasites that enter the host orally and which require activation by specific triggers in the intestinal environment may not experience these factors or the combination of factors that is necessary.

Even if the host provides an environment suitable for initial development incompatibilities may well arise at subsequent stages through nutritional inadequacies, or through incomplete stimuli for migrations and reproductive maturation. The eggs of the human *Ascaris, A. lumbricoides,* for example, can hatch in a variety of mammalian hosts because of the relatively low specificity of the intestinal signals required (mammalian body temperature, alkaline pH, dissolved CO_2 and a reducing environment). After hatching the larvae can migrate and reach the lungs but development after this point, and sexual maturation, occurs only in man. It follows from this that, in natural host–parasite relationships, the parasite must be precisely adapted to the structural and physiological conditions that characterize the host species. This adaptation, which develops over long periods of evolutionary change, is the basis for the phenomenon of host specificity, i.e. the restriction of parasites to particular species of hosts. In some cases the restriction is near absolute, as occurs with the human malaria parasites and certain of the human filarial nematodes. In other cases the restriction is extremely loose and parasites can undergo development in, and be transmitted between, a wide variety of hosts, as occurs with the nematode *Trichinella spiralis.* For the majority of parasites host specificity falls between these extremes and under natural conditions particular species are found in only a few species of hosts.

1.4 Acquired Resistance to Infection

In established host–parasite relationships, where natural resistance is low, the host can regulate the degree of infection to which it is subject only through the activities of its immune system, that is by developing an acquired resistance to infection. The degree to which such regulation is in fact operative, or indeed necessary, under natural conditions is an open question and one for which little evidence is available. It is conceivable that in the wild, rates of transmission are such that parasite burdens remain below the thresholds necessary for the stimulation or expression of immune responses. With protozoan infections, of course, this factor is then offset by the parasite's ability to reproduce within the host. Rates of transmission are determined by a number of environmental factors, of which host density is one of the most important. It is the alterations of these factors, which man imposes upon himself and his domestic animals, that lead to increased rates of transmission, increased prevalence and intensity of infection thus emphasizing the role of acquired immunity in control. Even where it is obvious that acquired immunity is necessary, the degree to which the host succeeds in regulating infection in this way is very variable. Many parasites have evolved successful means of evading the immune response that they evoke and some seem not to evoke protective responses at all. Others depend for their survival as a species on development and reproduction within individual hosts that are, for various reasons, incapable of developing or expressing an adequate protective immunity.

Implicit in the concepts of host specificity and of balanced relationships is the assumption that the ability of the host to control the parasite is never absolute. Several workers have put forward the concept that in evolution there is always a tendency towards a mutual adjustment between the two species, the parasite reducing its pathogenicity and immunogenicity so as to elicit weaker host responses, the host reducing its responsiveness so that parasite control is achieved without concomitant pathological change. 'Successful' parasites therefore tend to become harmless to the host. An example frequently cited in support of this concept is the relatively benign association of trypanosomes in game animals compared with the pathological consequences of infections in man. Whether this interpretation is of general applicability is open to question. Many associations are still remarkably pathogenic for the host, in others the host rapidly achieves control of the parasite. Although it seems self-evident that mutual adjustment is necessary for mutual survival there are many parasites, particularly those transmitted through food chains, for which death or incapacity of the host can only facilitate their own transmission. It is, in fact, likely that there is no single trend in the evolution of host–parasite relations and that a variety of endpoints may be achieved, however three factors in particular suggest that the host–parasite relationship is always a confrontation for survival. One is the variability within species of the mechanisms controlling natural and acquired resistance. This implies the operation of strong selective pressures from infectious organisms. The second is the very existence and complexity of the resistance mechanisms possessed by all animals, but particularly by vertebrates. It is hard to see why such elaborate devices should have evolved, and why they should have persisted, if they did not confer powerful selective advantages. The third is the evidence of substantial genetic variability within parasite populations, which attests to the effectiveness of selection pressures exercised by host resistance.

2

The Immune Response

Protection against Invading Organisms

The ability to discriminate between 'self' and 'not-self' is present throughout the animal kingdom and indeed may be seen as a precondition for the evolution of complex animal organization as we know it. Recognition of 'not-self' certainly occurs in the Protozoa, where it is used in the selection of food, of compatible mating types and, in parasitic species, of appropriate host cells. The importance of this ability, and its relevance for survival, increased enormously with the evolution of multicellularity and the associated increases in size and complexity. In multicellular organisms this ability has at least three major roles to play in preserving the integrity of the body:

(*a*) in minimizing the consequences of contact with related but foreign (allogeneic) organisms,
(*b*) in preventing the proliferation of mutant cells,
(*c*) in defence against invading pathogens.

The first of these is of significance only in primitive sessile animals, such as sponges and corals, in which contact, through growth, with other species is a regular occurrence. It is well known that these simple organisms possess efficient mechanisms of allogeneic recognition, capable of inducing destructive cytotoxic reactions and thus preventing intermixing of colonies. It is remarkable that these recognition mechanisms also show the property of short-term memory and enhanced effectiveness on re-presentation of the foreign stimulus. In higher animals recognition processes are primarily concerned with defence against mutant cells and against pathogens. The importance of these processes, and the complexity of the mechanisms concerned with their operation, increases with the cellular complexity of the animal, reaching a peak in the warm-blooded vertebrates, i.e. in the birds and mammals (Fig. 2.1).

In lower invertebrates recognition of not-self is limited mainly to the detection of foreignness in molecules presented at the surfaces of cells. Expression of effector mechanisms is also primarily a surface phenomenon, mediated almost exclusively by phagocytic cells. In vertebrates this basic ability is further elaborated, but is supplemented and overshadowed by the development of *adaptive immunity*, which allows a much greater sophistication and effectiveness in response. The improved capability stems from the evolution of a class of cells, the lymphocytes, whose

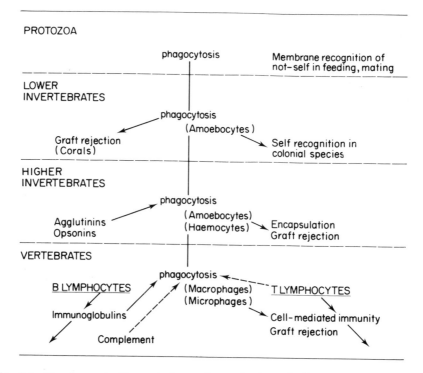

PROTOZOA

phagocytosis — Membrane recognition of not–self in feeding, mating

LOWER INVERTEBRATES

phagocytosis (Amoebocytes)

Graft rejection (Corals) — Self recognition in colonial species

HIGHER INVERTEBRATES

phagocytosis (Amoebocytes) (Haemocytes)

Agglutinins Opsonins — Encapsulation Graft rejection

VERTEBRATES

phagocytosis (Macrophages) (Microphages)

B LYMPHOCYTES — T LYMPHOCYTES

Immunoglobulins

Complement

Cell-mediated immunity Graft rejection

Fig. 2.1 Development of increasingly complex mechanisms of self–notself discrimination in animal evolution.

homologies in invertebrates are controversial. Among the many important advantages conferred by the adaptive immune response are:

(a) The ability to discriminate not only between self and not-self, but also among an enormous variety of not-self, foreign molecules (*antigens*).
[Although it is conventional to refer to foreign molecules an 'antigens', what is recognized as foreign is not the whole molecule but particular antigenic determinants or epitopes (discrete structural configurations) on that molecule. Complex molecules therefore present several antigenic determinants each of which may be recognized by the immune system. Strictly speaking, therefore, a complex molecule is equivalent to several antigens.]

(b) To retain long-term memory of foreignness and to respond more rapidly on subsequent contact (the *anamnestic response*).

(c) To produce large amounts of free receptor material (*antibody*) capable of combining with soluble or membrane-bound antigens.

(d) To interact with a number of other resistance mechanisms, including the ancestral phagocytic cells.

(e) To confer protection against infection upon offspring.

Phagocytic cells still play important roles in resistance against infection, through their participation in inflammatory reactions, but their activities in warm-blooded hosts are so inextricably linked with immune responses that it is difficult to conceive of active anti-parasite responses that do not have a major immunological component.

2.1 The Major Histocompatibility Complex

Implicit in the ability to recognize not-self is the recognition of self. This is an active process, i.e. it depends upon the presence of self molecules rather than the mere absence of not-self. A great deal is now known about the structure, production and control of such self markers, particularly in mammals. Their identification originated in experiments involving grafting of tissues between related and unrelated animals and for this reason they were described as *transplantation* or *histocompatibility* antigens. Their involvement in graft recognition and rejection clearly represents an unnatural situation and there has been much speculation about their natural functions. It is now recognized that these molecules play key roles in the immune response, but their original designations have been retained.

The results of the early transplantation experiments showed that there were both major and minor histocompatibility antigens, i.e. antigens evolving strong and weak rejection responses when tissues were exchanged between unrelated individuals. The gene loci coding for these antigens have been identified in several species but are most completely known in mice and men. In every species studied it has been found that the genes which code for the major histocompatibility antigens are grouped together on one particular chromosome, forming the *major histocompatibility complex* (MHC). The genes within the MHC are grouped closely together and thus appear to segregate in a simple Mendelian fashion. Recombinations between the genes do occur and can be produced readily using defined strains of mice.

In man the MHC is located on chromosome 6 and is known as the HLA (human leucocyte antigen) complex; in mice the MHC is located on chromosome 17 and is known as the H–2 (histocompatibility antigen 2) complex. The major regions of both MHC are shown in Fig. 2.2. Until recently the H–2 complex was more extensively subdivided, but it is now accepted that the many distinct functions formerly attributed to distinct regions of the complex represent different facets of a smaller number of identifiable regions.

One of the most striking features of the MHC is its extreme polymorphism. Each locus has many alleles and thus, in outbred populations, the chances of two unrelated individuals sharing an identical MHC haplotype (complement of loci) are very small indeed. Within inbred strains of animals, of course, each individual is effectively genetically identical and thus shares the same MHC haplotype. The availability of such animals, most particularly mice, and their suitability for genetic and immunological analysis has made it possible to explore the functions of the MHC in great detail.

MHC coded antigens are known to occur on a wide variety of cells, especially on lymphocytes. Not every cell expresses all MHC antigens equally strongly. In mice, for example, H–2K and H–2D antigens are widely distributed and function in allogeneic recognition, i.e. they are the major foreign not-self antigens recognized on cell membranes. H–2I region antigens (Ia antigens) occur primarily on lymphocytes and macrophages and have an important function in the cell–cell interactions that initiate and regulate immune responses (see Fig. 2.5).

One of the most important observations concerning the immunological functions of the MHC has been that the ability to make responses to particular antigens can be genetically determined and is associated with particular MHC-linked genes, the so-called *Ir* (immune-response) genes. Not all *Ir* genes are MHC-linked, but many are and their loci have been mapped within the I region. Controversy surrounds the precise manner in which *Ir* genes function. However evidence suggests an important role in determining the efficiency of antigen presentation between macrophages and lymphocytes, and the cooperative interactions between lymphocytes.

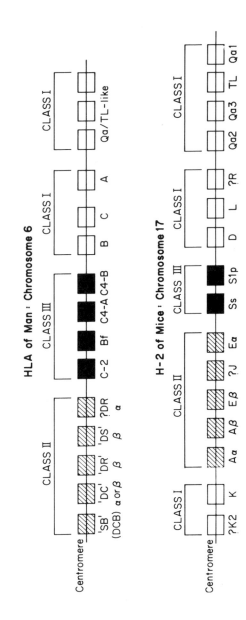

Fig. 2.2 The major histocompatibility complexes of man and mouse. The molecules coded for by the loci in the MHC fall into three major classes, Classes I, II and III. There are two functional groups of Class I molecules, the classical transplantation antigens expressed on almost all somatic cells, (HLA, B, C; H–2 K, D, L, and R), which are also involved in target cell destruction by cytotoxic T cells, and the lymphocyte differentiation antigens (Qa/TL). Class II molecules are expressed primarily on B cells and macrophages and are involved in antigen presentation. Class III molecules are components of the complement system and as such are functionally distinct from the rest of the MHC. In the mouse, immune response genes are predominantly located in the I region of the H–2 complex, i.e. in the region containing loci controlling Class II molecules. (taken from Robertson, 1982, *Nature*, **297**, 629.)

2.2 Lymphocytes

The basic patterns of lymphocyte development and differentiation are summarized in Fig. 2.3. In development, lymphocyte precursors arise from yolk sac cells and foetal liver, but subsequently all lymphocytes develop from stem cells that originate

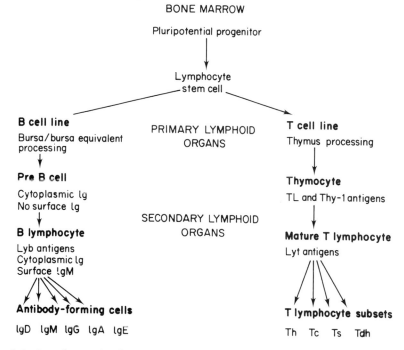

Fig. 2.3 Lymphocyte development and differentiation.

in the bone marrow. Two major pathways of differentiation are then followed, each involving one of the major primary lymphoid organs. The two pathways lead to the production of two classes of lymphocytes, one concerned primarily with cell-mediated immune responses and helper function, the other with humoral, i.e. antibody-mediated responses. In the first pathway, precursor cells pass to the thymus and there undergo proliferation and maturation to become thymus-dependent or T lymphocytes. Mature T cells leave the thymus and pass to the secondary lymphoid organs, the spleen and lymph nodes, forming part of the lymphocyte population located in these organs or recirculating around the body. The second pathway of lymphocyte differentiation is seen most clearly in birds, where it involves a defined primary lymphoid structure, the bursa of Fabricius, which is not present in mammals. Lymphocytes differentiating in this organ are referred to as B (= bursa dependent) cells and like T cells, become distributed among the secondary lymphoid organs. The homologous population in mammals are also referred to as B cells, but their site of differentiation is controversial. Evidence has been presented which implicates gut-associated lymphoid tissue (GALT) or bone marrow as the mammalian bursa equivalent, but there is no coherent picture for the entire class.

During their differentiation T and B cells acquire surface molecules that serve as characteristic markers and which play important roles in their cellular functions (Table 2.1). These markers coexist with molecules coded for by genes within the

Table 2.1   Surface membrane markers found on mouse T and B lymphocytes.

	T	B		T	B
H–2 Class I (K/D)	+	+	C3b receptor	–	+
H–2 Class II (1)	–	+	IgFc receptor	–	+
Thy 1	+	–	Lectin receptors		
Ly t	+	–	e.g. Con A	+	–
Ly b	–	+	PHA	+	±
Ig	–	+	PWM	+	+
			Endotoxin (LPS) receptor	–	+

MHC. Both T and B cells carry receptors capable of combining specifically with antigen, the progeny of each clone of cells carrying receptors for one particular antigen. The nature of the receptor differs between the two classes of cells. In B cells the receptor is immunoglobulin, in T cells the precise identity of the receptor is unknown. T and B cells also differ in other membrane characteristics, in particular in their abilities to combine with lectins, substances of plant origin which recognize specific sugars in glycoproteins. Exposure of lymphocytes to lectins triggers transformation and cell division. Measurement of cellular responses to such mitogens, together with identification of surface receptors, can be used as convenient means of identifying and differentiating between the two populations.

The secondary lymphoid organs have a characteristic structural organization (Fig. 2.4) within which T and B cells are distributed in precisely defined regions. Lymph and lymphocytes flow through these organs, draining specific parts of the body and returning to the general circulation via the thoracic duct. Lymphocytes also enter the spleen and lymph nodes from the blood. The cells pass through the specialized endothelium of the post-capillary venules, move through the organ and then rejoin the efferent lymph. The functional signficance of this structural organization and pattern of circulation is that it allows the organs to 'sample' the lymph and to bring antigens into contact with lymphocytes. Retention and presentation of antigen is the function of dendritic cells, specialized cells of the phagocytic series. The consequence of antigen presentation to lymphocytes bearing the appropriate receptors is a sequence of proliferation within the germinal centres and paracortical areas. The cells produced are then released into the circulation and become distributed around the body. Distinct circulatory patterns exist, with lymphocytes originating from the GALT homing back to the intestine and other mucosal surfaces, those from other lymphoid organs homing to the rest of the body. In a resting condition, recirculating lymphocytes are predominantly small, non-dividing cells. After antigenic stimulation, substantial numbers of large dividing cells (lymphoblasts) and their immediate progeny are found in the thoracic duct lymph.

In man there are a number of well-defined, genetically-determined deficiencies in lymphocyte development and function. Patients suffering from these abnormalities may lack normal T-cell function (e.g. the DiGeorge and Wiskott–Aldrich Syndromes) or B-cell function (e.g. congenital agammaglobulinaemia) and be severely immunodeficient. Study of such conditions has contributed greatly to an understanding of lymphocyte activity in relation to resistance to infection. Congenital deficiencies also occur in experimental animals, the best known and most useful of which is the athymic condition in nude mice and rats. Lymphocyte deficiencies can readily be produced experimentally in otherwise normal animals. T-cell deprivation can be achieved by thymectomy, thoracic duct drainage, or by treatment with

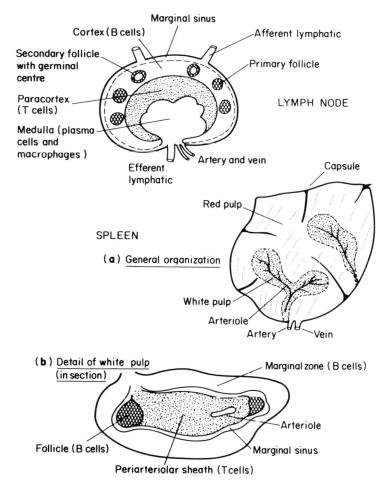

Marginal sinus

Cortex (B cells)

Afferent lymphatic

Secondary follicle
with germinal
centre

Primary follicle

Paracortex
(T cells)

LYMPH NODE

Medulla (plasma
cells and
macrophages)

Efferent
lymphatic

Artery and vein

Capsule

Red pulp

SPLEEN

(a) General organization

White pulp

Arteriole

Artery

Vein

(b) Detail of white pulp
(in section)

Marginal zone (B cells)

Arteriole

Follicle (B cells)

Marginal sinus

Periarteriolar sheath (T cells)

Fig. 2.4 Diagrammatic representations of the gross architecture of lymph node and spleen, with distribution of T and B lymphocyte areas.

anti-thymocyte serum. B-cell deficiency can be induced by treatment with anti-Ig sera during neonatal life.

2.3 Recognition of Antigen and Initiation of the Immune Response

Stimulation of the immune response requires that antigenic material is processed by accessory cells and presented to lymphocytes in an appropriate form and manner. Direct contact of antigen with lymphocytes can in fact induce unresponsiveness. Presentation is achieved by macrophages and related phagocytic cells. These are responsible for taking up antigen after it has entered the body, processing it, and then re-presenting antigen on their surface membranes in close association with MHC-coded (Ia) molecules. In this form antigen is available for recognition by T cells carrying the complementary receptors. The precise entity recognized by the T cell is controversial and two main concepts exist:

(*a*) that there is separate recognition of the antigenic determinant and the associated MHC-coded molecule – simultaneous recognition of both being essential for T-cell activation.

(*b*) that the antigenic determinant and the MHC molecule together form a new structure and it is this that is recognized as a single entity by the T cell.

Whichever is true, it is important to realize that recognition for foreignness is possible only in the context of a self molecule. This has particular implications when considering immunity against intracellular parasites (Chapter 4).

After T-cell triggering transformation of the lymphocyte occurs, the cell becoming larger and entering a division cycle. It is now known as a T lymphoblast and its behaviour is profoundly influenced by a variety of soluble mediators released from macrophages (e.g. Interleukin 1) and other T cells (e.g. Interleukin 2). Proliferation continues under the stimulus of these factors, increasing the number of cells carrying specificity for the antigen concerned. The fate and function of these cells varies considerably, depending upon a number of factors present at the time of antigen stimulation. Some cells revert to the small resting phase as memory cells, thus providing the cellular basis for enhanced secondary responsiveness. Others function as helper or as suppressor cells. Each function is the property of distinct subsets of T cells, identified by the possession of characteristic surface membrane markers (Fig. 2.5). Helper cells may interact with other T cells in the production of cytotoxic (killer) cells, or of cells capable of initiating delayed hypersensitivity reactions. They also interact with B cells to initiate formation of antibody. In each case, interaction with other lymphocytes, or other cell types, involves the synthesis and release of mediators known as lymphokines.

2.4   Antibody Production and Immunoglobulins

Not all antibody production is dependent upon prior help from T cells. Certain molecules, the thymus-independent antigens, can bypass the requirements for macrophage and T-cell processing and stimulate B cells directly. It is characteristic of such antigens, many of which are carbohydrate, that they possess serially-repeated antigenic determinants. This fact has led some workers to the conclusion that thymus-dependent antigens require processing (focussing) so that a similar repetitive structure may be presented to B cells.

The interaction between T helper cells and B cells again involves both antigen and MHC-coded molecules. It is not always necessary for there to be physical contact between the cells for this interaction to be successful. Soluble factors, having both antigenic and MHC specificity, may help B cells just as effectively. Following triggering, the B cell enlarges, enters a division cycle and becomes a B lymphoblast or plasmablast. The progeny of these dividing cells may either become small memory cells or remain large, differentiate into plasma cells and secrete immunoglobulin (Ig). Plasma cell precursors have Ig present intracellularly before they express Ig at the cell surface. In most cases the Ig formed initially is IgM, but there is then a switch to other isotypes (classes of Ig) under the control of T cell help. Each plasma cell normally secretes Ig specific for only one antigenic determinant, and this specificity remains despite the changes to different isotypes.

2.4.1   Immunoglobulins

Development of the ability to produce Igs can be seen as one of the major steps in the evolution of the adaptive immune response. It represents a facet of the vertebrate response which is essentially without parallel in the invertebrates. An

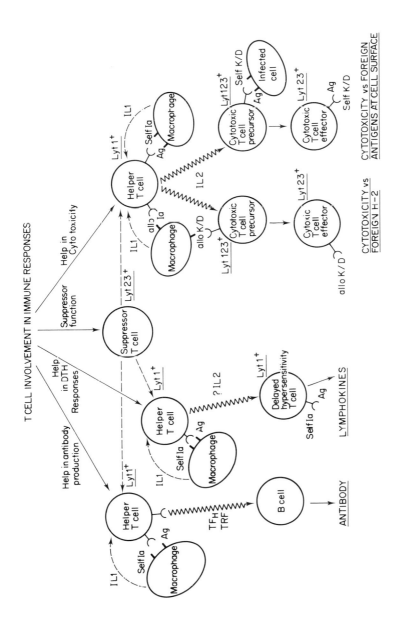

Fig. 2.5 Generalized scheme to show the roles played by mouse T cells in immune responses. T cells are shown with the Lyt phenotype characteristic of the subset concerned, although in every case there is some controversy over the precise phenotype concerned. Ag = Antigen, Ia self = Class II H–2 coded molecules of self origin, IL1 = Interleukin 1, a T-cell activating factor released by macrophages, IL2 = Interleukin 2, a T-cell growth factor released by stimulated T cells (possibly a distinct subset), K/D self/allo = Class I H–2 coded molecules of self or foreign (allogeneic) origin, TF_H = T helper factor, TRF = T cell replacing factor, ⊻ = T cell receptor

instructive way of thinking of these molecules is to view them as cell surface receptors, produced in excessive quantities and released into the circulation. Here they can fulfill their recognition function at some distance from the source of production. This makes possible the localization of organs in which plasma cells can be concentrated, without losing the ability to provide the whole body with efficient protection.

Recognition and combination with antigens is the primary function of Igs, but combination is then followed by a variety of biological effects, the nature of which depends upon the isotype involved. In order to explain this point more fully it is necessary to understand in outline the structure of Ig molecules and to be aware of the differences which exist between isotypes.

The basic structure of Ig can be seen in the IgG molecule, which is composed of two identical light chains and two identical heavy chains, held together by a number of disulphide bonds (Fig. 2.6). Each chain consists of regions where amino acid sequences are constant between different molecules of the Ig class (the constant regions) and regions where the sequences are variable. The variable regions lie at the

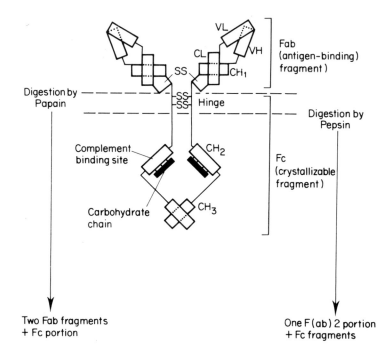

Fig. 2.6 Representation of an IgG_1 molecule, based on the Edelman and Porter model. The molecule is formed of 2 identical light chains (MW 25 kD) and 2 identical heavy chains (MW 50 kD) held together by disulphide bridges. The light chains are folded into two domains VL and CL, the heavy chains into four domains VH, CH_1, CH_2 and CH_3, and all except CH_2 are arranged in pairs held together by non-covalent forces. The amino acid sequences of the domains are variable (V) or constant (C) and the antigen binding sites are associated with hypervariable regions in the VL and VH domains. Digestion by proteolytic enzymes breaks the molecule into a variety of fragments. The Fab fragments contain the active antigen-binding sites, the Fc portion determines the biological characteristics of the molecule. (Based on Marquart and Deisenhofer, 1982, *Immunology Today*, **3**, 160.)

N-terminal ends of the light and heavy chains and contain within them areas where there is hypervariability in sequences.

The Ig molecule can be split, by papain digestion, into three units, two Fab fragments, consisting of variable and constant regions of the light and heavy chains, and one Fc fragment, which consists of the constant regions of the heavy chains. Antigen specificity resides in the Fab fragments and is associated with the hyper-variable regions. These form structural configurations which are complementary to those of the appropriate antigenic determinants. The Fc fragment (so called because it can be crystallized) determines the biological properties of the Ig molecule and these are characteristic for each isotype (Table 2.2). Activation of

Table 2.2 Biological characteristics associated with immunoglobulin isotypes.

	IgM	IgG	IgA	IgE
Fixation of complement				
Classical path	+	+	−	−
Alternative path	−	−	±	−
Binding to amine-				
containing cells	−	+ (some sub-classes)		+
Binding to macrophages				
and granulocytes	−	+	−	−
Cross placenta	−	+	−	−
Secreted across				
mucous surface	+	−	+	−

complement, which is discussed further below, is dependent upon the properties of a specific region (domain) of the Fc fragment, the configuration of which alters after antigen-antibody combination. Activation is most efficient with IgM, because the pentamerous structure of the molecule results in fixation of a proportionately greater number of complement molecules than occurs with monomeric Igs.

With the exception of IgD, all Igs can readily be identified in blood and tissue fluids. IgM and IgA can also be actively secreted across mucosal membranes and thus form the major Igs in the normal intestinal lumen. Secretion occurs across the epithelial cells of the mucosae and, in the case of IgA, across cells lining bile ducts, and requires the addition to the Ig molecule of a secretory piece. This both facilitates trans-epithelial passage and protects intramolecular linkages from the action of enzymes. In this way the functional life of the Ig is prolonged in the proteolytic environment of the intestine.

2.4.2 Immunoglobulin Function

Combination of Ig with antigens may have many different consequences. When antigen is soluble it may be precipitated through cross linkage and thus rendered both biologically inactive (e.g. toxins neutralized, enzymes inactivated) and made available for phagocytosis. Combination with particulate antigen likewise may result in agglutination, leading to inactivation (e.g. organisms become non-infective) and phagocytosis. Attachment of IgG antibody to particulate antigens or antigen-coated surfaces, the process of opsonization, facilitates phagocytosis if the object is of a suitable size, or cell attachment if phagocytosis is impossible. Where the object or surface is parasitic, then attachment may be followed by release of lysosomal enzymes or other cytotoxic factors causing the destruction of the parasite. This is a particular example of antibody-dependent cell-mediated cytotoxicity (ADCC) in which many cell types may participate, both lymphoid and myeloid. Such cells are often collectively termed killer cells, but the term is usually restricted to a subset of lymphocytes which are neither T nor B cells but possess Fc receptors. (Natural Killer (NK) cells are also lymphoid, but are cytotoxic in the absence of Ig.) In both phagocytosis and ADCC the antigen and the cell are linked by means of antibody combined with the former and Fc receptors on the latter. Phagocytes and other cells may similarly be armed for interaction with, and destruction of, invading organisms by the binding of immune complexes to their cell membrane. The complex allows specific adherence by means of free antibody combining sites in the complex. ADCC by eosinophils can also be achieved via interaction between specific IgE on a parasite surface and IgE Fc receptors on the cell membrane (see Fig. 2.7).

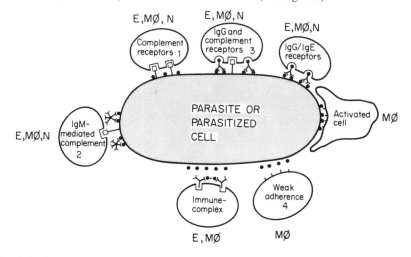

Fig. 2.7 Summary diagram showing the variety of interactions that are possible between the surfaces of parasites or parasitized cells and cells of the myeloid series, i.e. eosinophils (E), macrophages (MØ) and neutrophils (N). The interaction may lead to phagocytosis if the parasite is small or ADCC if it is large, or there may be no measurable effect. (1) activation of complement by the alternative pathway, (2) fixation of complement by IgM molecules, (3) fixation of complement by IgG molecules, (4) weak adherence may occur between glycoproteins and sugar receptors. (Based on Roitt, 1980, *Essential Immunology*, Blackwell Scientific Publications, Oxford.)

Interaction of antigen with IgG and IgM molecules makes available on the Fc region a site to which the initial components of complement can attach. Complement is the name given to a complex of nine proteins present in serum. When complement becomes attached (fixed) to an antigen–antibody complex there follows a series of reactions, each component of complement acting enzymatically to release subsequent components in a cascade fashion. Activation of complement can also occur in the absence of immune complexes, the cascade being triggered by the presence of soluble factors or surfaces of infectious organisms. The stages involved in the classical and alternative pathways of complement activation are shown in Fig. 2.8.

Many of the complement components are biologically active. They mediate chemotaxis of inflammatory cells and immune adherence of phagocytes, they cause release of histamine and bring about vasodilation, and the end products of the

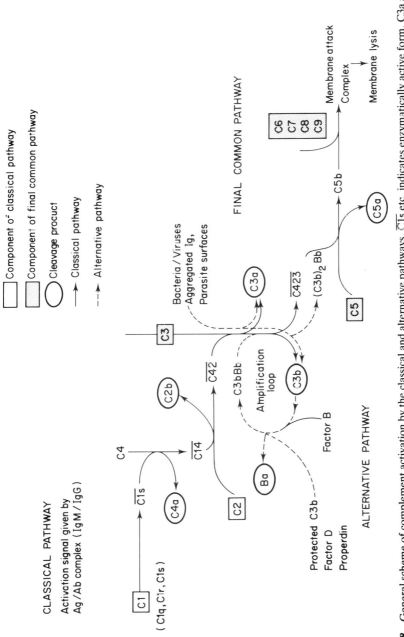

Fig. 2.8 General scheme of complement activation by the classical and alternative pathways. $\overline{C1s}$ etc. indicates enzymatically active form. C3a and C5a are biologically active, with inflammatory and chemotactic properties, C3b attaches to cell membranes and promotes phagocytosis. Inactivators have been omitted.

cascade exert a powerful lytic action on cell membranes. Three of the most important products in the context of parasite immunity are C3b, which readily attaches to cell membranes and thus promotes adherence of cells bearing C3b receptors, C3a and C5a which have chemotactic and anaphylatoxin (histamine-releasing) activity. Phagocytic cells may bear receptors for both IgG Fc and C3b, so that opsonization of parasites by this isotype is doubly effective in causing cell adherence and phagocytosis. Destruction of antibody-coated cells and organisms is also brought about by non-phagocytic mechanisms (ADCC) involving C3b–C3b receptor interactions and a variety of cells (see summary Fig. 2.7).

Two Ig isotypes, namely IgE (= reaginic antibody) and certain subclasses of IgG, can bind through the Fc region to receptors present on the surfaces of mast cells and basophils, cells specialized for the production and release of a variety of potent biologically-active mediators including the vasoactive amines. When cells with these Igs bound to their surfaces are subsequently exposed to the eliciting antigen, the Igs are cross-linked. This cross-linkage results in release of mediators, which then initiate the tissue inflammatory reactions of immediate hypersensitivity, best known in examples of allergic reactions such as hay-fever.

2.5   Interactions between Lymphocytes and Myeloid Cells

The vertebrate immune response to infection is an integrated response, involving not only the cells of the immune system proper, i.e. the lymphocytes and their products, but also a variety of other cells, the myeloid cells, which are likewise derived from stem cells originating in the bone marrow. Within this category three distinct cells lines can be considered, the macrophage-monocyte series, the granulocytes, and the amine-containing cells.

2.5.1   Macrophage–Monocyte Series

These cells form part of what was formerly referred to as the reticulo-endothelial system, but is now described more appropriately as the mononuclear phagocyte system. The earlier name emphasized the fixed phagocytic cells of the body, e.g. those in the spleen and liver: the latter emphasizes the morphological and functional characteristics of both these fixed cells and the mobile population dispersed throughout the tissues. Monocytes circulate in the blood and are the immediate precursors of the macrophages. Macrophages represent a direct link with the scavenging phagocytic cells possessed by more primitive animals, and still have an important role in this respect. However, in vertebrates they also play a vitally important part in the induction, regulation and expression of immune responses. This is related to their capacity to process and present antigen, to release a variety of soluble factors (monokines) and to interact with the surfaces of malignant cells or invading organisms. Many aspects of macrophage function are intimately connected with the presence on the cell membrane of MHC coded molecules and a variety of receptors. Over 15 such receptors are now defined, including the IgG Fc and C3b receptors discussed above which play an important role in mediation of phagocytosis.

Phagocytic activity is enhanced and directed by lymphokines released from T cells and by factors present in invading pathogens. Thus, in response to macrophage activating factor from T cells, macrophages become more motile, phagocytose or adhere more readily and digest more efficiently when material is taken into the phagolysosomes. In this activated state macrophage function may be expressed non-specifically, i.e. although activation follows a specific stimulus, such as an immune response to organism A, the cells will then readily phagocytose and destroy any other organisms (B, C, D, etc) accessible to them. Specificity in macrophage function can be achieved by arming with antibody, immune complexes or with specific arming factor released from T cells. The armed and activated macrophage is then able to participate in a variety of specific effector functions, including ADCC. The ability of the cells to damage and kill organisms during contact, or after phagocytosis, resides in their production and release of lysozyme, lysosomal hydrolases and other factors, as well as a variety of oxygen metabolites, including singlet oxygen ($^1O_2$), hydrogen peroxide (H_2O_2) and superoxide (O_2^-) (Table 2.3). Production of these oxygen metabolites is associated with a burst of oxygen consumption, the oxidative burst, linked to the process of phagocytosis, and is more efficient in activated cells.

Table 2.3 Factors released from macrophages which interact with other components of the immune and inflammatory systems.

Lysozyme	α−2 macroglobulin
Neutral proteinases	Complement components
Acid hydrolases	Interferon
Interleukin 1	Prostaglandins
Oxygen metabolites	Leukotriene C
α−anti trypsin	Fibronectin

2.5.2 Granulocytes

Eosinophils and neutrophils, present both in blood and in body tissues, are characterized by polymorphic nuclei and prominent cytoplasmic granules. Neutrophils are sometimes referred to as microphages and have as a primary function the phagocytosis and destruction of microorganisms. They possess both Fc and C3b receptors and, as a result, their efficiency in phagocytosis is enhanced when specific antibody is bound to the organism or if the surface of the organism itself activates complement. After uptake, the organism is killed in the phagolysosome by lysozyme, lysosomal enzymes, cationic proteins and oxygen metabolites, and some of these factors may also be released by exocytosis into the extracellular environment. Neutrophils are positively attracted by C3a, one of the products of complement activation, as well as by lymphocyte and mast cell factors. This chemotaxis plays an important role in directing defensive responses. Unfortunately this attraction also occurs wherever antigen–antibody complexes form, and the accumulation of neutrophils, together with the extracellular release of their enzymes, contributes to tissue inflammation.

The role played by eosinophils has been obscure, although their association with the inflammatory responses and parasitic infections has been known for many years. Clarification of their function has come largely from recent studies of their *in vitro* interactions with helminths. The characteristic granules of these cells contain a variety of hydrolytic enzymes, including peroxidases, and prominent central bodies which contain cationic proteins. It has been shown that the eosinophil membrane bears both Fc and C3b receptors, which make it possible for the cell to adhere to target surfaces coated with antibody or complement components. An important finding is that Fc receptors exist for IgE as well as for the customary IgG. Adherence is followed by release from the granules of enzymes, the major basic protein of the granule core, and other factors which readily damage cell membranes. The production and activities of eosinophils are regulated by T lymphocytes through lymphokines and, additionally, by complex interactions with amine-containing cells.

The latter release a powerful eosinophil chemotactic factor (ECF–A), which attracts eosinophils into sites of amine release and may increase their receptor density. Eosinophils in turn release factors which counteract the activity of released amines.

2.5.3   Amine-containing Cells

Within this category are included the mast cells and basophils, two cell types with many functional similarities, but with some basic differences. Basophils circulate in the blood and occur in the tissues; mast cells occur only in the tissues and, in rodents at least, form two distinct populations, one restricted to mucosal surfaces, the other distributed in connective tissues. The myeloid origin of basophils and their relation to granulocytes have never been in question; the demonstration that mast cells are similarly derived is very recent. Both cells are heavily granulated and contain a variety of extremely potent mediators, including histamine, 5-hydroxytryptamine (serotonin), heparin, enzymes and chemotactic factors. The membranes of both cells carry receptors for the Fc regions of IgE and particular IgG sub-classes. Crosslinking of membrane bound Ig by antigen triggers exocytosis of the granules and release of their contents. Amine-containing cells are typically associated with immediate hypersensitivity reactions (see below) but it is becoming accepted that they may also be involved in a number of immune-mediated events and evidence has been presented recently to show that degranulation can also be induced by T cell products. The interactions between parasites, myeloid cells and lymphocytes are summarized in Fig. 2.9.

2.6   Hypersensitivity

Under certain conditions, the normal secondary response to contact with a previously experienced antigen is associated with exaggerated reactions that may result in tissue damage. Some are rapid, explosive responses, others are delayed in development, all are referred to as hypersensitivity reactions. Such reactions were originally categorized by Coombs and Gell into Types I, II, III and IV (Fig. 2.10). The first three are sometimes collectively referred to as the immediate hypersensitivity reactions because of the speed of onset, but this term is commonly restricted to Type I, which is dependent upon interactions between reaginic antibodies and amine-containing cells. Type II reactions are antibody-dependent cytotoxic phenomena (ADCC) and Type III are antigen-antibody complex-mediated reactions. Type IV are delayed-type hypersensitivity reactions (DTH) that are distinctive not only in their slower time course, but also in their primary reliance upon T cells rather than upon antibody. Types I, III and IV are considered briefly below.

2.6.1   Immediate Hypersensitivity

The cellular and antibody components of this reaction have already been described. Reactions are triggered when antigens cross-link antibody molecules bound to receptors on the surfaces of mast cells or basophils. Their effects are entirely due to the release of potent mediators which bring about immediate physiological changes such as increased contractility of smooth muscle and increased permeability of blood vessels and epithelial membranes. In severe cases the reaction is a generalized anaphylaxis with systemic involvement. More often the reaction is localized, affecting parts of the body that meet environmental antigens, e.g. skin and mucous membranes. An important consequence of mediator release and increased permeability is the escape of plasma and cells into inflamed tissues or into the lumen of organs such as the intestine. The reactions are modulated by factors released from other cells, notably eosinophils, which rapidly inactivate the mediators responsible.

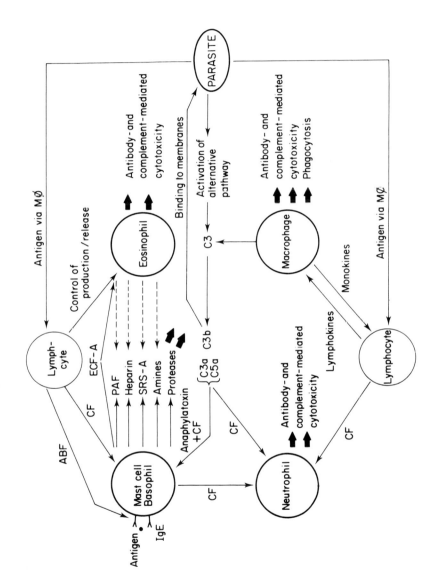

Fig. 2.9 Schematic representation of the interactions between lymphocytes and myeloid cells and their relationship to protective antiparasite responses. ABF = T cell produced, antigen-binding factor, C3 etc. = complement components, CF = chemotactic factor, ECF–A = eosinophil chemotactic factor of anaphylaxis, PAF = platelet activating factor, SRS–A = slow reacting substance of anaphylaxis. ──→ signifies factors released by cells, ── signifies inactivating factors released by eosinophils, signifies anti-parasite directed responses. (Based upon Klein, 1982. *Immunology. The Science of Self – Nonself Discrimination.* John Wiley & Sons.)

26

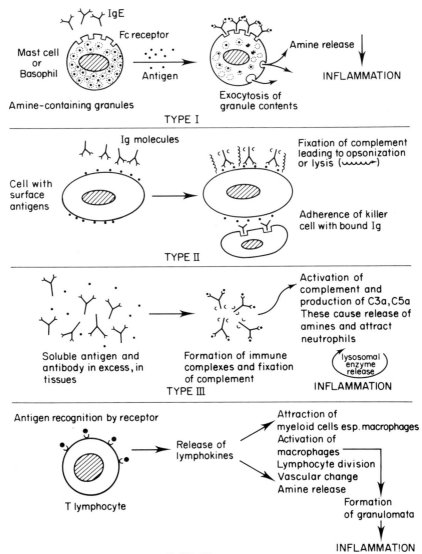

Fig. 2.10 Summary of hypersensitivity reactions.

Type I: Anaphylactic (Immediate), usually initiated by IgE antibody but can involve sub-classes of IgG.

Type II: Antibody-dependent cytotoxic, resulting in lysis of cells by complement or by killer cells.

Type III: Complex-mediated, shown here as an Arthus reaction in tissues, but occurring in other forms, e.g. serum sickness, where complexes formed in antigen excess circulate and become deposited.

Type IV: Delayed, shown here in relation to granuloma formation, but occurring in other forms, e.g. the cutaneous basophil hypersensitivity (Jones–Mote) reaction and the generation of killer T cells. (Based on Taussig, M.J., 1979. *Processes in Pathology*, Blackwell Scientific Publications, Oxford.)

Eosinophils are in fact selectively recruited to sites where Type I reactions are in progress through the release of chemotactic factors.

2.6.2   Immune Complex-Mediated Hypersensitivity

Fixation of complement by antigen–antibody complexes results in the liberation of components which, in combination, lead to the generation of inflammatory responses. C3a and C5a cause release of histamine, thus increasing vascular permeability locally, they also attract neutrophils, which phagocytose complexes and in so doing release a variety of factors, including enzymes, that damage surrounding tissues. If uncontrolled, inflammation intensifies in a vicious circle. When immune complexes are formed in antibody excess they are readily precipitated and complex-mediated damage is localized – the Arthus type reaction. In antigen excess, complexes remain soluble and circulate around the body before being deposited in various tissues, which then become the focus of inflammatory lesions.

2.6.3   Delayed-Type Hypersensitivity

DTH is a correlate of the cell-mediated immunity that protects against an number of intracellular infections, notably those of bacterial origin. In its classical form, e.g. in the response to tuberculosis, it is initiated by a subset of T cells which, after recognition of antigen, release lymphokines that attract, localize and activate macrophages at the site of antigenic stimulation. Characteristically the inflammatory site becomes populated by mononuclear cells, i.e. lymphocytes and macrophages, rather than polymorphonuclear cells. Neutrophils appear only in the initial stages, eosinophils may appear later. The development of cytotoxicity in T cells, as is seen during graft rejection, can also be considered a form of DTH, and is closely linked to the appearance of armed macrophages, which are also cytotoxic in this situation. A specialized form of DTH is the Jones–Mote reaction, or cutaneous basophil hypersensitivity, in which, as the name implies, inflammatory sites in the skin are infiltrated by basophils. This reaction has recently received a great deal of attention and appears to be an important defensive response against ectoparasitic arthropods (Chapter 9).

Although each type of hypersensitivity reaction has been considered separately, it is likely that there is a complex interplay between them in any hypersensitivity response. Certainly Type I reactions are now thought to form an important component in the development of Type III and Type IV, primarily by facilitating extravasation and accumulation of effector cells at sites of injury and antigen deposition. This aspect is clearly relevant to anti-parasite responses and will be discussed in greater detail in later chapters.

3

Experimental Immunoparasitology

3.1 Parasite Maintenance
3.2 Antigenic Complexity
3.3 Identification and Measurement of Immunity

Immunity to parasites, in the sense of protection from infection, or from the consequences of infection, has been recognized empirically for a very long time, even though the underlying causes have not been understood. As can be seen from early texts on this topic, anti-parasite immunity was originally approached very much in the same terms as classical anti-microbial immunity. However, it is now clear that many significant differences exist, in part related to the greater size and complexity of parasites. Immunoparasitology as a distinct discipline has been a comparatively recent development and it is only in the last decade or so that substantial progress has been made. On of the most important factors in encouraging work in this field has been the World Bank/W.H.O. programme of research into parasitic diseases of man. This has stimulated a much greater awareness of the problems caused by parasites and has encouraged cooperation between parasitologists and immunologists in searching for improved methods of immunologically-based control. An essential part of this cooperation has been the investigation of fundamental aspects of the immunological relationship between hosts and parasites.

Parasites present a number of difficulties for the experimentalist concerned with analysis of immunity. These can be considered under three headings:

(*a*) parasite maintenance in the laboratory,
(*b*) antigenic complexity,
(*c*) identification and measurement of immunity.

3.1 Parasite Maintenance

Immunological analyses of *in vivo* responses are most conveniently carried out using well-defined experimental animals, in which variables can be fully controlled. Many parasites of medical or veterinary importance (e.g. human malarias, filarial nematodes) show rigid host specificity and cannot readily be passaged in laboratory hosts. The choice is then between studying the parasite in its natural host, with the attendant difficulties in experimentation, or using related parasites which can be maintained in the laboratory, but which may not always be entirely appropriate as model systems. A third possibility is to use *in vitro* maintenance. Some significant progress has been made in this field and the availability of techniques for long-term culture of *Plasmodium falciparium* and bloodstream form trypanosomes has vastly increased research potential. However, such techniques are available for relatively few species, the restrictions being particularly acute with helminths. Some, e.g.

schistosomes, larval nematodes, can be kept successfully in short-term cultures, but few can be maintained for extended periods or taken through their complete life cycles. Of equal significance is the problem of modelling *in vitro* the conditions associated with the expression of immunity in the host. For some parasites, e.g. gastro-intestinal species, where immunity is expressed primarily in expulsive mechanisms, it is unlikely that this will ever be achieved.

3.2 Antigenic Complexity

Animal parasites are complex organisms and may have complex developmental cycles. As a result they present both host and immunoparasitologist with a battery of antigenic material, much of which is undefined. There are, therefore, difficulties in relating particular components of a parasite to the generation of immune responses, and of differentiating between antigens which elicit protective responses and antigens with no apparent role in resistance, i.e. between 'functional' and non-functional antigens.

A useful, though arbitrary distinction has been made between antigens which are associated with structural components of a parasite (structural antigens) and those that are released as a result of metabolic processes (metabolic or excretory–secretory (ES) antigens). Many attempts have been made to immunize animals against infection using homogenates of parasite material. Although some have been successful, the majority have not, even though infection with the parasite generates an effective immunity. As a consequence, attention has been directed to antigens associated with, or released from, the living parasite as an essential requirement for successful immunization. The nature of such antigens has been defined in certain species (see succeeding chapters) but in general, relatively little progress has been made in this field.

Another area of difficulty with parasite antigens is the lack of information concerning their origin and biological function, or the ways in which they may be presented to the host (Fig. 3.1). Structural antigens, other than those which form components of surface membranes, will normally not be available to the host's immune system whilst the parasite is alive. Metabolic antigens, once released, may diffuse rapidly from the vicinity of the parasite. In the first case, the host may recognize the antigens after the death of some of the parasites, but effector mechanisms will be unable to interact directly with them in living parasites. In the second, recognition and effector interactions may occur at some distance from the parasite and thus be relatively ineffective. It should be clear from this that, in analysing immune responses which interact in a direct manner with living parasites and which can damage them, it is natural to look for antigens present at their surfaces, i.e. at the immediate host-parasite interface. As will be discussed later, however, not all immune responses that are effective against parasites achieve this effectiveness in a direct fashion. The generation of inflammatory changes plays an important role in protection against many parasites and in such cases a wide variety of metabolic antigens may serve to initiate and focus the protective response.

With intracellular parasites, appearance of antigen at the cell surface may be an important requirement for the stimulation and expression of immunity. As has been discussed in Chapter 2, under these circumstances antigens will be recognized in the context of self (MHC coded) molecules. A good example of such immune responses is seen with intra-macrophage parasites of the genus *Leishmania*. The converse of this is that if self-molecules are absent or sparse, as on red blood cells, immunogenicity is reduced even though, as with malaria parasites, antigens may be expressed at the red cell surface. Many intracellular organisms are most vulnerable to immune attack

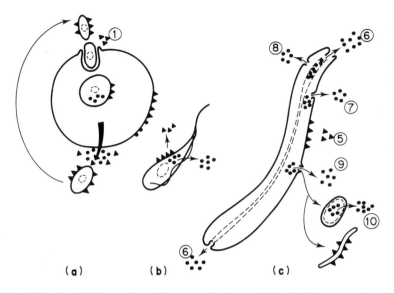

Fig. 3.1 Ways in which parasite antigens may be presented to the immune system of the host. ▼ ▼ represent surface (membrane) antigens; ● ● represent internal antigens.
(a) Intracellular protozoa with extracellular invasive stages. (1) Antigens are present on the surface of invasive stages and may be released on entry. (2) Antigens from the intracellular stages appear on the membrane of the host cell and are released (3) when the cell ruptures to release the next generation of invasive stages.
(b) Extracellular protozoa. Antigens are presented on the surface. Both surface and internal antigens are released into the host tissues.
(c) Helminth parasites. (5) Antigens are presented on the surface and are released into the host tissues. Internal antigens are released during feeding (6), excretion (7), moulting (8) and reproduction (9). Reproductive stages may continue to present antigens when retained in the body (10).

when they are released into the extracellular environment. Under these conditions their surface antigens are exposed directly to antibodies, and in consequence the organisms may be agglutinated, phagocytosed or lysed. Protozoa that live extracellularly lack the protection of a host cell and are always exposed directly to effectors of the immune system. Some, notably the African trypanosomes, solve this problem by their powers of antigenic variation. These parasites are among the few for which there exist detailed molecular analyses of antigens and the genetic mechanisms controlling their production.

Helminths, as metazoan parasites, are larger and have a more complicated level of organization than protozoans. They therefore show a greater antigenic complexity. There are, however, sufficient examples in which particular antigenic fractions have been shown to have a major role in stimulating protective immunity to encourage the view that this complexity does not create an impossibly difficult situation for analysis. Platyhelminth worms, such as schistosomes, have bodies that are covered by a potentially vulnerable, plasma membrane-bounded surface. They release a wide variety of metabolic antigens, but the major antigens that are relevant to protective immunity are undoubtedly those located at the surface of the body. Nematodes, on the other hand, have a tough outer cuticle that certainly confers a degree of protection against immune attack. Despite earlier views to the contrary, it is now known that the cuticular surface is both antigenic, i.e. will bind antibodies, and is immunogenic, i.e. will stimulate antibody production. Antigen turnover and release into the surrounding environment has also been demonstrated. With certain species, and particularly with larval stages, immune attack directed against surface antigens can result in damage and death. The relevance of surface antigens to immunity is more apparent with tissue-dwelling worms, such as filarial nematodes, than it is with intestinal worms. In the latter, immunity seems more dependent upon antigens released during feeding, excretion, moulting and reproduction. In the case of feeding, inactivation of digestive enzymes by combination with antibody, though it occurs at some distance from the worm, may very effectively reduce viability and therefore lead to parasite elimination.

The antigens responsible for immunity to arthropods are more easily identified than in other parasites. This is because they are almost entirely associated with feeding, and particularly with secretion of saliva. Unlike helminths, therefore, the origin of the antigens and their function in the life of the organisms are more immediately apparent. It is unlikely that immune interaction with these antigens is itself harmful to the arthropod. Indirect consequences of such interaction, such as the generation of inflammatory changes are likely to be the effectors of resistance, and these may act in ways as non-specific, but as effective, as scratching.

3.3   Identification and Measurement of Immunity

Infection with parasites and exposure to their complex antigens, generates a complex immune response. This may be measured using a variety of the conventional immunological tests that determine levels of antibody activity or cellular sensitization. Such tests, however, frequently provide little or no correlation with the degree of protective immunity that the host may possess. It must therefore be concluded that many of the responses that are elicited by infection are irrelevant to the continued well-being of the parasite. They may represent responses to antigens that are not critical to survival, or responses that do not interfere sufficiently seriously with the functional integrity of critical antigens. Protective immunity can often be measured only by parameters that can be correlated directly with normal parasite development, such as growth and reproduction, or by determing the actual numbers of parasites present. Although these parameters allow resistance as such to be assessed with some accuracy, they are, at best, crude indicators of the underlying immune responses, if only because there will often be a significant time lag between the onset of a response and the detection of measurable changes in the parasite population. Identification of the immune effector mechanisms underlying and responsible for resistance can only come from experimental manipulations of host and parasite, using both *in vivo* and *in vitro* approaches. There are, in the immunoparasitological literature, many papers describing immunological responses in infected hosts, and many describing the expression of resistance in terms of its effects against the parasite concerned. In relatively few have the two phenomena been clearly interrelated.

Immunoparasitology therefore presents a number of peculiar problems to the research worker concerned with untangling the complex interrelationships between host and parasite. Despite these problems there are a number of fruitful analyses of immune responses to parasites and these will form the subject matter of the chapters which follow.

4

Intracellular Protozoa

Survival within Cells

4.1 *Plasmodium* and Malaria
4.2 *Leishmania* and Leishmaniasis

Several species of Protozoa live as intracellular parasites, occupying a variety of cells within the body of the host. Included among these species are a number which are of major medical and veterinary importance and responsible for widespread disease (Table 4.1).

Table 4.1 Major intracellular protozoa of man and domestic animals.

Parasite	Cell	Disease	Host
Babesia spp.	RBC	Piroplasmosis (Red Water Fever)	Cattle
Plasmodium spp.	RBC, Hepatocytes	Malaria	Man
Eimeria spp.	Intestine, Liver	Coccidiosis	Fowl, Sheep, Cattle
Toxoplasma gondii	Macrophages and many others	Toxoplasmosis	Man
Leishmania spp.	Macrophages	Leishmaniasis (Kala Azar, Oriental Sore)	Man
Trypanosoma cruzi	Macrophages, Muscle	Chagas' Disease	Man

Life within cells poses certain problems for the protozoan, such as recognition and penetration of the correct cell, and transmission between hosts. At the same time it confers many advantages, of which protection from potential immune effectors is certainly one and these advantages have, in evolution, outweighed the difficulties inherent in this mode of life. Recognition and penetration of suitable cells is dependent upon complex membrane interactions and will be discussed again later. Transmission between hosts is achieved in many cases by arthropod vectors; in species which parasitize intestinal cells (e.g. *Eimeria*, *Toxoplasma* in the final host) the normal mode of transmission is via a resistant cyst. The manner in which the intracellular location influences the immunological interactions between host and parasite is determined by the nature of the cell occupied and will be discussed primarily in relation to *Plasmodium* and *Leishmania*.

4.1 *Plasmodium* and Malaria

Malaria ranks as one of the commonest and most important parasitic diseases. It is estimated that some 1000 million people are at risk from infection and 200 million are actually infected. In Africa, for example, infection leads to 1 million deaths annually, the majority of deaths occurring in children. The distribution of infection is determined by the vector arthropods, species of anopheline mosquitoes, and major foci occur in Africa, India, S.E. Asia, Central and S. America. Despite intensive programmes of vector control, which have been successful in some countries, there has been no significant global reduction in the extent of malarial infection. Indeed, in certain countries, after a period of control there have been serious resurgences, arising from breakdown of control measures and the emergence of insecticide and drug resistance. In India the annual number of cases in 1962 was 100 000, but this has risen again to 10 million in recent years.

Man is the intermediate host of *Plasmodium*, the sexual stages of the life cycle taking place in the body of mosquito (Fig. 4.1). Infection is initiated by the bite of an infected mosquito and the injection into the bloodstream of sporozoite stages contained in the insect's saliva. The sporozoite enters hepatocytes of the liver shortly after injection, (possibly via Kupffer cells) undergoing growth and asexual reproduction (schizogony) to form a large pre-erythrocytic schizont. Rupture of the infected cell releases thousands of merozoites, which then penetrate red blood cells (RBC) to initiate the erythrocytic cycle. After a period of growth, during which the parasite passes through the ring and trophozoite stages, there is schizogony and production of the erythrocytic schizont, with division of cytoplasm and nucleus to form a relatively small number (32 or less) of merozoites. The infected cells then burst, releasing merozoites, and repeated cycles of schizogony and RBC infection ensue, so that a high proportion of available RBC may become infected.

Growth of the parasite in the RBC is fuelled by intake and digestion of RBC cytoplasm. Haemoglobin is digested, to obtain amino acids, but the haem is stored in the form of an insoluble pigment. When the infected RBC bursts, pigment and other metabolic products are released into the circulation, inducing a number of changes in the host, of which fever is the most characteristic. In the human malarias there is synchrony of schizont formation and RBC rupture, and this is responsible for the regular and repeated bouts of fever which are almost diagnostic of the infection.

After repeated cycles of asexual division there is a switch to the sexual phase of the cycle. Merozoites invade RBC and produce male or female gametocytes rather than a further generation of schizonts. No further development can occur unless the cells containing gametocytes are taken up by a suitable mosquito. Production of male gametes and fertilization of the female gamete occurs in the stomach of the mosquito. The motile zygote then penetrates the stomach wall and forms an oocyst on the outer lining. Within the oocyst there is repeated division to produce large numbers of sporozoites and these eventually move anteriorly in the insect to enter the salivary gland.

In two of the species of human malarial parasites (*P. falciparum* and *P. malariae*) the duration of infection is determined by the duration of the asexual schizogonic phase in the RBC, and this may be very prolonged in the latter species. In *P. ovale* and *P. vivax* prolonged infections arise from relapses, i.e. from re-invasion of RBC by merozoites released from liver schizonts that have remained dormant.

The pathological consequences of malarial infection are primarily associated with the destruction of RBC, which can lead to anaemia and vascular collapse. In *falciparum* malaria, the most dangerous form, there is an additional primary cause of pathology. Cells containing schizonts are sequestered in capillaries of internal organs.

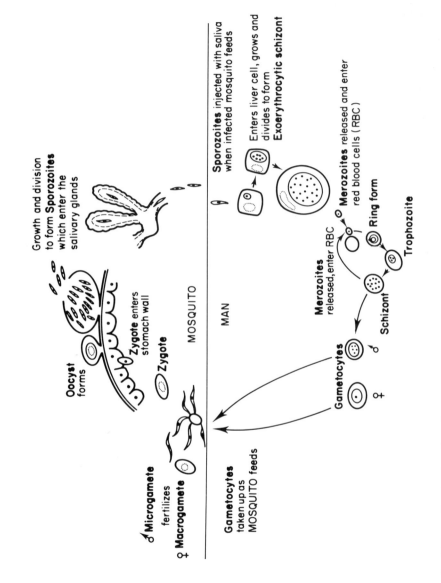

Fig. 4.1 Life cycle of *Plasmodium* in mosquito and man.

If the brain is involved, the damage caused by blockage of capillaries can lead to the fatal condition known as cerebral malaria. Other pathological manifestations arise as secondary consequences of infection, for example the nephrosis that follows immune complex-mediated damaged to the kidney.

4.1.1 Immunity to Malaria

Despite the fact that infection exposes the immune system to a very considerable antigenic challenge, there is in Man at best only an incomplete immunity to the parasite and this wanes rapidly in the absence of re-infection. That immunity does develop can be deduced from the fact that, in areas where malaria is endemic, adults survive with intermittent appearance of parasites in the blood (parasitaemia) whereas children are heavily infected and suffer extensively from clinical disease. Babies under the age of 3 months are relatively resistant to infection and this is attributable to transfer of maternal immunity. More direct evidence for immunity can be gained from *in vitro* experimentation, e.g. by studying the effects of serum taken from patients living in endemic areas upon the growth and division of malaria parasites in cultures of infected RBC (Fig. 4.2). The mechanisms through which protection can be expressed and factors which operative against effective resistance have been explored in great detail using a variety of experimental model systems in primate and rodent hosts (Table 4.2) and *in vitro* studies using human materials. Five important concepts have emerged from this work:

(*a*) natural resistance
(*b*) species specificity
(*c*) stage specificity
(*d*) antigenic variation
(*e*) immune-suppression

Natural Resistance

It is well known in man that susceptibility and resistance to malaria are influenced by several factors that have nothing to do with immunologically-mediated responses to infection and which may affect the parasite at distinct phases of its development. Entry of merozoites into the RBC depends upon a complex process following interaction between molecules on the parasite surface and receptors on the RBC membrane. Contact between the two leads to temporary attachments forming and then movement of these zones of attachment over the parasite until it is completely enclosed by the RBC membrane and internalized within the cell. Certain genetic variants of RBC lack the appropriate receptor molecules and, as a result, are not penetrated by merozoites. This has been most clearly shown for merozoites of *P. knowlesi*, which are unable to enter cells lacking Duffy blood group antigens. *P. knowlesi* is the monkey equivalent of the human *P. vivax* and it is almost certain that the absence of *vivax* malaria from areas of West Africa can be explained by the fact that the population contains a high proportion of Duffy negative individuals.

Natural resistance may also arise after merozoites have entered RBC. If there are unfavourable factors present in the environment provided by the RBC cytoplasm, then the growth and division of the parasite may be hindered. As a result the host may suffer a much less serious infection. The best known example of such an effect is seen in individuals heterozygous for the gene determining the formation of sickle-cell haemoglobin (HbS), in which there is a substitution of valine for glutamic acid in the β chain of the molecule. Cells containing HbS provide a relatively poor environment for growth and development of *P. falciparum* and the host is thereby protected

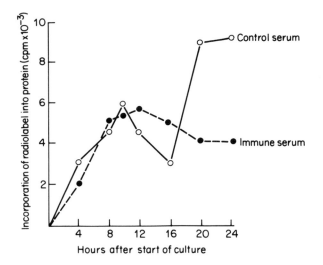

	Time 0 h		Time 16 h		Time 24 h	
	Cont	Imm	Cont	Imm	Cont	Imm
Parasites 10^{-4} RBC	78	78	268	93	249	83
% rings	0	0	86	64	90	56
% trophozoites	36	36	–	–	–	–
% schizonts	63	63	8	20	–	–
% abnormal forms	1	1	6	16	8	44

Fig. 4.2 Effect of control and immune human sera on the development of *Plasmodium falciparum* in *in vitro* culture. Schizont-stage parasites were subcultured into media containing control or immune sera. Development was followed by examination of samples at intervals for stages present in RBC and by measuring incorporation of (^{14}C) isoleucine into the protein fraction of each culture. (Data from Phillips *et al.*, 1972, *Parasitology*, **65**, 525.)

Table 4.2 Non-human species of *Plasmodium* used for experimental studies of malarial immunity in primate and rodent hosts.

Host	Parasite
Primate	*P. cynomolgi, P. inui, P. knowlesi*
Rodent	*P. berghei, P. chabaudi, P. vinckei, P. yoelii*

against the serious consequences of this form of malaria. In the homozygous state the sickle cell condition is invariably fatal and there is little doubt that the persistence and high frequency of the HbS gene in endemic areas results from the major selection pressure exerted by *P. falciparum* on the human population. A number of other haemoglobin mutants and RBC abnormalities (e.g. thalassaemias and G6PD deficiency) are likewise maintained in populations by this selection pressure.

Species Specificity of Immunity

This aspect of acquired resistance has been most thoroughly studied in model systems, but there is good clinical evidence, and some supporting experimental data, that in man, immunity against one species of human malaria does not confer protection against the others; this has been confirmed using human malarial infections in primates. Primate malarias themselves generate species-specific immunity and there is only limited cross immunity between the four rodent malarias most commonly used in experimental studies (Table 4.3). Two important conclusions stem from these observations. Firstly, that there are species-specific, protection-inducing antigens, and secondly, that protective immunity involves recognition of these specific antigens by immunologically specific effector mechanisms. Although

Table 4.3 Cross immunity in rodent malarias to the erythrocyte stages of infection. (Data from Cohen and Lambert. In *Immunology of Parasitic Infections* (eds. Cohen & Warren) 1982, p. 422.)

Species used for challenge	Species used for immunization		
	P. chabaudi	P. berghei	P. yoelii
P. chabaudi	+	−	
P. berghei	−	+	±
P. yoelii		+	+
P. vinckei	+	−	−

these conclusions may appear self-evident, they lead to the inference that cross-reacting antigens, and effectors which recognize such antigens, play no part in protective immunity. It should therefore be possible, by elimination, to identify those antigens and effectors which might be relevant.

Stage Specificity of Immunity

Not only is acquired immunity specific for the species of malaria involved, but it also operates specifically against particular stages in the life cycle. Thus, immunity generated experimentally by vaccination with erythrocytic stages has no effect upon the initial sporozoite-induced stages of infection and vice versa. Again this phenomenon is indicative of stage-restricted antigens and it is clear that there must be significant differences between the immune mechanisms which are effective against the various extracellular stages of the cycle, i.e. the sporozoite and merozoite, and those effective against the intracellular stages. Each will be considered separately.

SPOROZOITE In naturally-acquired infections the sporozoite represents a transient phase and appears to generate little protective immunity, even though anti-sporozoite antibodies are present in sera of patients from endemic areas. Nevertheless it is now well established that the sporozoite possesses antigens capable of eliciting protective immunity and exposure to radiation-attenuated sporozoites has been used to generate an effective resistance against homologous challenge both in man and in experimental animals. Immunization results in the formation of anti-sporozoite antibodies which react primarily with antigens present at the sporozoite surface (Plate 4.1). Incubation in immune serum *in vitro* results in the formation of a

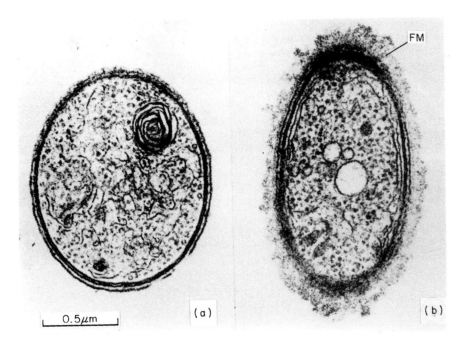

Plate 4.1 Surface antigens of malarial sporozoites: effect of incubation in immune serum. (**a**) TEM through sporozoite of *Plasmodium berghei* incubated in normal mouse serum. (**b**) TEM through sporozoite of *P. berghei* incubated in immune mouse serum. The surface of the parasite is covered by a thick coat of fibrillar material (FM). (Photographs from Nussenzweig *et al.*, 1978. In: *Rodent Malaria* (eds Killick-Kendrick & Peters), Academic Press, p. 248, by permission of the authors and publishers.)

circum-sporozoite precipitate which appears then to be cast off as long filamentous threads, possibly as a result of capping (Plate 4.2). Such incubated sporozoites lose their infectivity and it has been assumed that this is because their ability to recognize and invade RBC has been destroyed.

Recent studies with *P. berghei*, using monoclonal antibodies produced by hybridomas derived from the spleen cells of sporozoite-immunized mice, have identified a major surface antigen with a molecular weight of 44 kD. This antigen is present only on the mature salivary-gland sporozoites and is absent from subsequent erythrocytic stages of the parasite. Passive transfer of the IgG_1 monoclonal which recognized this antigen gave mice a high degree of protection against homologous challenge, even when as little as 10 μg of antibody was used. During *in vitro* neutralization experiments it was found that Fab fragments of the IgG_1 monoclonal were as effective as the intact Ig molecule in abolishing infectivity of the incubated sporozoites. It could therefore be concluded that the antibody was in some way blocking the ability of the parasite to recognize or to penetrate the target cell, rather than initiating a secondary effector activity against the sporozoite. It would seem obvious that anti-sporozoite immunity should be achieved most efficiently by antibody, but it has been shown that mice treated from birth with anti-μ chain antisera (and thus incapable of antibody production) can still respond to vaccination with irradiated sporozoites and resist a challenge with normal sporozoites. The cellular basis of this form of immunity is unknown.

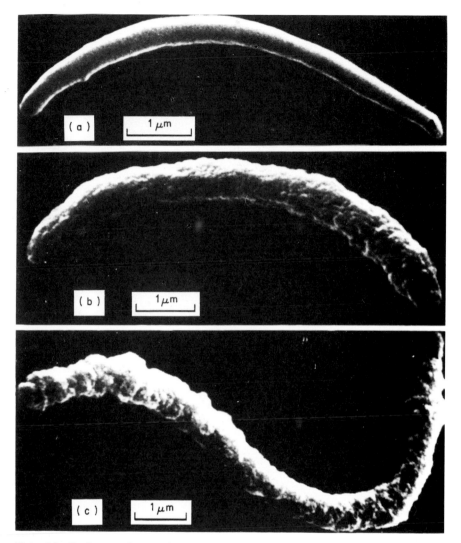

Plate 4.2 Surface antigens of malarial sporozoites: formation of circum-sporozoite precipitate (CSP). (**a**) SEM of sporozoite of *Plasmodium cynomolgi* incubated in normal monkey serum. The surface of the parasite appears smooth. (**b**) and (**c**) SEM of sporozoite of *P. cynomolgi* after incubation in immune monkey serum. The surface outline is irregular and the parasite appears much thicker. In (**c**) the deposited material extends posteriorly for some distance, forming the tail-like CSP. (Photographs from Cochrane *et al.*, 1976, *Journal of Immunology*, **116**, 859, by permission of the authors and publishers).

MEROZOITES   These are the second extracellular phase of the cycle, and must survive in the face of developing immunity if the infection is to continue. The degree of effective immunity against the erythrocytic cycle varies considerably between species. In infections in man, for example, immunity develops only slowly, whereas in rodent infected with *P. berghei* a sterile immunity, i.e. one in which no parasites remain, may develop quite rapidly. This situation may reflect the differences between a host-parasite relationship with a long evolutionary history of mutual adaptation and an abnormal relation in which the balance is very much in favour of the host.

Use of merozoite preparations to stimulate immunity has been effective with a variety of malarial species, but has been most extensively studied in primate malarias. Isolated merozoites lose their infectivity after a short period and can therefore be used in vaccines without any additional form of inactivation. Injection of merozoites of *P. knowlesi* with a variety of adjuvants effectively protects rhesus monkeys against the challenge infections that are lethal to immunized controls (Fig. 4.3). Immunization does not protect completely against infection, but in those animals in which infection does develop parasitaemias are low and of short duration. Merozoite vaccines have also been shown to give protection against infection with *P. falciparum* in *Aotus* monkeys.

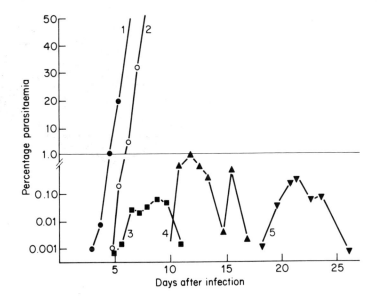

Fig. 4.3 Course of an infection with *Plasmodium knowlesi* in Rhesus monkeys. Monkeys 1 and 2 were un-immunized controls and died within 10 days. Monkeys 3, 4 and 5 had been immunized by injection of merozoites in Freund's complete adjuvant. Parasitaemia is shown on a log scale to accommodate the extremes recorded in control and immunized animals. (Redrawn from Mitchell *et al.*, 1975, *Immunology*, **29**, 397.)

The extracellular position of the merozoite makes it a vulnerable target for immune effector mechanisms, particularly for antibodies, and indeed there is a considerable body of evidence implicating humoral mechanisms in anti-merozoite immunity. For example, immunity can be passively transferred, and such transfer has been achieved in man; conversely infections are more severe in animals rendered incapable of antibody production. The action of antibody can be studied *in vitro*, using continuous culture of infected RBC, in which the regular cycles of growth, schizogony, merozoite release and cell invasion occur quite normally. Studies made using a variety of species, including *P. falciparum*, *P. knowlesi* and *P. berghei* have shown

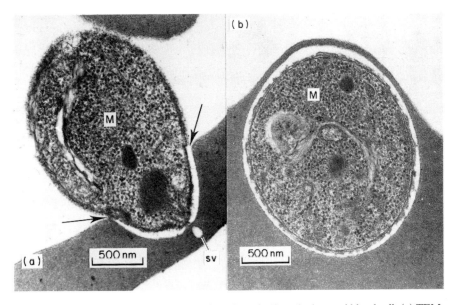

Plate 4.3 Entry of merozoite of *Plasmodium knowlesi* into the host red blood cell. (a) TEM showing invagination of red cell surface and attachments between rim of invagination and merozoite surface coat (arrowed). A subsidiary vacuole (sv) is forming at the base of the invagination. M = merozoite.(b) TEM of merozoite (M) within vacuole inside red cell. (Photographs from Bannister *et al.*, 1975, *Parasitology*, **71**, 483, by permission of the authors and publishers.)

that antibody blocks merozoite entry into RBC (Plate 4.3). This presumably is a consequence of parasite agglutination or of antibody binding to surface antigens and thereby interfering with the interaction of merozoite molecules with RBC receptors. Blocking can be achieved with the F(ab)2 fragment of the appropriate IgG_1 antibody (i.e. with the divalent antigen-binding fragment) and is complement independent. Passive transfer of monoclonal antibody specific for the merozoite stage of *P. yoelii* has shown that it is also possible to block infection *in vivo*, and it is reasonable to assume that similar anti-parasite mechanisms may be involved, although under these circumstances antibody might additionally opsonize merozoites for phagocytosis. Some evidence that this is the case is provided by experiments using transfers of hyper-immune serum, which showed that protection was reduced in recipients that had been splenectomized.

Merozoite surface antigens involved in protective immune responses have been identified using the techniques of surface labelling and immune precipitation of solubilized fractions. The precision of identification has been increased by the availability of monoclonal antibodies. In *P. knowlesi* a major antigen of molecular weight 250 kD has been identified and it has been shown that antibodies recognizing this antigen will agglutinate free merozoites and block invasion of RBC. It has been possible to locate the mouse monoclonal binding to this antigen by using a ferritin-labelled anti-mouse Ig and the results shown that the antigen is distributed over the whole surface of the merozoite. Antigens of similar molecular weight have been identified on merozoites of *P. yoelii* and antibodies directed against these antigens likewise block cell invasion. There is also evidence that merozoite antigens of much lower molecular weight (65 kD) may contribute to the stimulation and expression of protective immunity. Antibodies to such antigens correlated well with immunity to *P. knowlesi* in naturally-infected animals.

SCHIZONT-INFECTED RBC   It is a reasonable assumption that the schizogonic stages of the life cycle are protected by virtue of their intracellular position (Plate 4.4) and there is experimental evidence to support this assumption. Antigens present on merozoites are also found in earlier schizogonic stages, but whereas antibodies to these antigens may agglutinate and opsonize free merozoites, they have no effect upon the intracellular stages. *In vitro* studies with T helper cells reveal a similar picture, in that helper activity is stimulated by free parasites but not by intact parasitized cells. An additional protection provided by life within the RBC is derived from the paucity of MHC-coded antigens on the RBC membrane. Such antigens are essential not only for the cellular recognition of foreign molecules at cell surfaces, but also for the expression of cytolytic function of effector cells. There is no evidence for any lymphocyte-mediated cytotoxicity against infected RBC. However the degree of protection afforded by the intracellular habit is only relative and the host is capable both of agglutinating parasite-infected RBC and of killing parasites within them.

Several studies have shown that there are malarial antigens present on the surface of infected RBC and present in the serum of infected hosts. Labelling experiments indicate that surface antigens originate primarily from the developing parasites within the cell, although it is not fully understood how transfer to the surface takes place (Fig. 4.4). Antibodies which react with these antigens also precipitate antigens

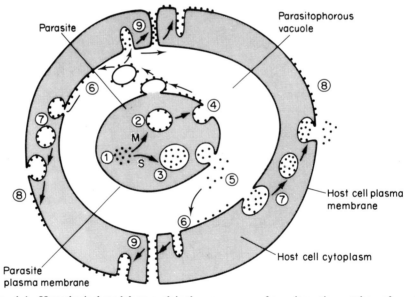

Fig. 4.4 Hypothetical models to explain the appearance of parasite antigen at the surface of malaria-infected red blood cells. Two pathways are shown one (M) involving membrane-bound antigen, the other (S) involving soluble antigen. Antigen is synthesized (1) and inserted into membranes of endoplasmic reticulum or Golgi vesicles (2) or contained in vesicles (3). In both, antigen is carried to the parasite surface and either fused with the plasma membrane (4) or released (5). Transfer to the membrane of the parasitophorous vacuole then occurs (6). Exocytosis of vesicles carries antigen to the outer plasma membrane of the host cell (7, 8), or antigen may be transported through the formation of temporary channels (9). (Based on Howard, 1982, *Immunological Reviews*, **61**, 77.)

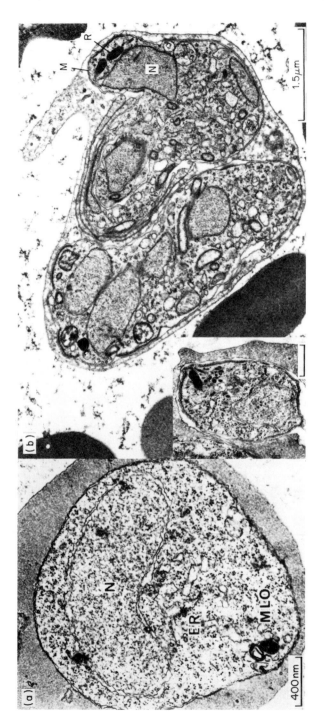

Plate 4.4 Intracellular stages of *Plasmodium yoelii* in the red blood cells of a mouse. (**a**) TEM showing young trophozoite with nucleus (N), endoplasmic reticulum (ER) and multilamellate organelle (MLO). (**b**) TEM showing young schizont with immature buds of merozoites (M) showing developing rhoptries (R) and migrating nuclei (N). Insert shows a mature merozoite in an older schizont (bar = 250 nm). (Photographs by courtesy of Dr R.E. Sinden.)

present in the ring, trophozoite, schizont and merozoite stages. In *P. falciparum* and other species it is known that infection of the RBC is associated with parasite-induced structural changes, some gross, others more subtle and affecting molecular components of the membrane. With *P. falciparum* there is production of knob-like extensions of the cell membrane, and parasite-derived polypeptides are present within these knobs. Presumably such alterations are minimal during early intra-erythrocytic development, but increase as the parasite matures and may then render the parasite-RBC complex vulnerable to host responses. Infection with *P. knowlesi* elicits antibodies capable of reacting with the surface antigens of schizont-infected cells. This interaction can be measured *in vitro* by agglutination of infected RBC, but there is little correlation with immunity. *In vivo*, antibody interaction may facilitate uptake of infected RBC by phagocytic cells or may interfere with passage of metabolites across the cell membrane.

Components of Protective Responses

The relative importance of individual components of the immune response in protection against malarial parasites is very difficult to assess. It is clear that immunity is T-cell dependent and that antibodies play a significant role, e.g. in blocking penetration of cells, and in agglutination/opsonization of infected RBC. The effectiveness of the humoral arm was demonstrated in the now classical experiment of Cohen, who showed that transfer of immunoglobulins from adults immune to malaria into infected children was followed by a rapid fall in parasitaemia. Nevertheless there is experimental evidence that antibodies are maximally effective when other host responses are also operative, for example when phagocytic cell activity is increased. Conversely, antibody is less effective is splenectomized animals. It is generally assumed that macrophages of the liver and spleen play an important role in clearing parastized RBC from the circulation, but there is some controversy over the mechanisms by which this is achieved. Prior opsonization of cells would appear essential, but is has also been claimed that increased uptake of infected RBC may result from alterations in the deformability of the cell and also reflect the large increase in spleen size (splenomegaly) that accompanies infection.

Immunity to malaria can be transferred adoptively by lymphocytes and in some cases (e.g. *P. berghei* in rats) adoptive transfer has proved more effective than passive transfer of serum. In general, however, despite variations between systems, transfers of B lymphocytes, or mixed populations of B and T cells, have given the best results and this reinforces the importance of antibody in immunity. It has been suggested that T cells may play a role in immunity other than that of helping production of antibody. Among those that have been proposed are direct cytotoxicity and induction of delayed hypersensitivity. Antibody-dependent lymphocyte-mediated cytotoxicity has been described using cells and serum from patients infected with *P. falciparum* and has been recorded in experimental systems. However, attempts to demonstrate a direct (antibody-independent) cytotoxicity have been largely unsuccessful. Classical DTH reactions have been elicited using parasite antigen in both human and experimental malarias. The *in vivo* correlate of DTH which may be relevant to immunity to infection would probably be T cell-mediated activation of macrophages, but at least one worker has excluded this possibility in rodent malarias on the grounds that immunity shows a high degree of species specificity, whereas protection mediated by activated macrophages should be non-specific. In opposition to this view is the elegant demonstration that mice rendered B-cell deficient (by neonatal injection of anti-μ chain sera) can be immunized against species such as *P. berghei* by immunization with irradiated sporozoites, or after chemotherapeutic cure of a primary infection, and thereafter remain resistant to challenge even though they are incapable of signficant antibody production.

Evidence for a direct effect of immunity on parasites within RBC has come from work with rodent malarias, with *P. knowlesi* in vaccinated monkeys and with *P. falciparum* in *in vitro* culture. During *in vivo* infections it has been observed that, at the times when parasitaemia reaches a peak, so-called 'crisis-forms' appear in the parasite population. In these the parasite is seen as a densely-staining, compact body and evidence suggests that the organisms are degenerating. Crisis forms appear rapidly in animals that have been injected with immuno-stimulants such as BCG or *Corynebacterium parvum* before infection. It has been suggested that the effector responsible for parasite killing is the release from macrophages, or possibly NK cells, of short-range factors capable of interfering with nutrient transport into the host cell, or of crossing the RBC membrane and acting directly. A number of candidate factors have been implicated, including interferon, but it is perhaps more likely that products of the oxidative burst associated with phagocytosis or cytolysis may be involved. The action of these factors, which are rapidly inactivated, would require RBC and macrophage (or NK cell) to be in close proximity and this is most likely to occur during circulation of blood through the spleen or liver. Studies with *P. falciparum* in continuous *in vitro* culture have shown that antibodies can exert effects upon the intracellular stages by interfering with transport of metabolites. In cultures exposed to immune serum parasite growth was retarded, reproduction during schizogony was reduced, and there was a general similarity to the crisis forms described *in vivo*.

Antigenic Variation

Malarial infections, particularly those established in natural hosts, are characterized by chronicity, with parasitaemias recurring at intervals after the initial patent parasitaemia has been controlled. In some species, notably *P. vivax*, recurrent parasitaemias are true relapses, the new erythrocytic cycles being initiated by merozoites released from latent exo-erythrocytic schizonts in the liver. In other species recurrent parasitaemias are recrudescences, derived from the multiplication of pre-existing erythrocytic stages. In laboratory models there is some evidence that recrudescence follows a decline in effective immunity, but a more significant factor in certain cases is the existence of antigenic variation, each recurrent parasitaemia representing a population that is antigenically distinct from the preceding population and thus is less well controlled by the host. Such variation was first described for *P. berghei* in mice and is now known to occur in *P. chabaudi*, *P. cynomolgi* and *P. knowlesi*; it probably also occurs in *P. falciparum* (Figs 4.5 and 4.6).

Compared with antigenic variation in trypanosomes little is known of the capacity of individual invasive stages (sporozoites or merozoites) to express a repertoire of variation or of the molecular basis underlying variation. In *P. knowlesi*, variation during chronic infections is relatively easily identified using the antibody-induced agglutination of schizont-infected RBC. During infection each recrudescence is associated with a distinct variant which stimulates the production of a specific agglutinating antibody, but which is not agglutinated by antibodies to earlier variants. The agglutinating antibodies themselves have no *in vivo* protective function, but there is, in addition, production of opsonizing antibodies, also variant specific, which are parasiticidal. It has been concluded that the agglutinating antibodies actively induce variation, thus allowing the parasite to survive even though protective opsonizing antibody is produced. Unlike trypanosomiasis, malarial recrudescences are eventually well controlled by the host, and the cross immunity between variants which has been described may be a contributory factor.

Variation in *P. chabaudi* has been detected directly by measuring the degree of immunity transferred against recrudescent populations by immune sera taken from mice after earlier parasitaemias. In these experiments the starting inoculum was a

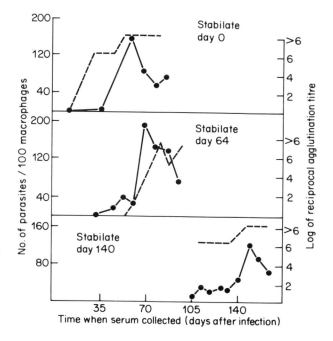

Fig. 4.5 Antigenic variation in *Plasmodium knowlesi*. Serum was taken from a chronically-infected monkey at intervals after infection and tested for activity against stabilates of the parasite collected at three time points during infection. Activity was measured by agglutination of schizont-infected cells (– – – – –) and opsonization by uptake of infected cells by macrophages. (●———●) (Redrawn from Brown & Hills, 1974, *Transactions of the Royal Society of Tropical Medicine and Hygiene,* **68**, 139.)

mosquito-passaged and cloned population. This was used to ensure a high degree of uniformity in the parasites and to reduce the possibility that recrudescence occurred from multiplication of antigenically-distinct forms present initially.

Immune Suppression

It has been known for more than 20 years that malaria infections in man can be associated with depressed responsiveness to unrelated antigens. This was shown originally by measuring the antibody responses of infected and uninfected children to vaccination with tetanus toxoid. Later studies extended the observations to responses against *Salmonella typhi*, but demonstrated that cell-mediated responses to purified protein derivative (PPD), *Candida* and streptococcal antigens were normal. Paradoxically, malarial infection is also associated with increased synthesis of immunoglobulin, particularly IgM and IgG. Clinically-immune West Africans produce about seven times as much IgG per day as do uninfected Europeans, and the level of synthesis falls markedly after anti-malarial drug treatment. It has been suggested that these increased levels of Ig are the result of a polyclonal activation of B cells, and that much of the Ig is not specific for malarial antigen.

Detailed analyses of malaria-induced immunosuppression have been undertaken with laboratory models, and a number of relevant points have been established. Direct evidence has been obtained that a mitogenic material is released from parasites during *in vitro* culture and this mitogen is thought to act directly on B

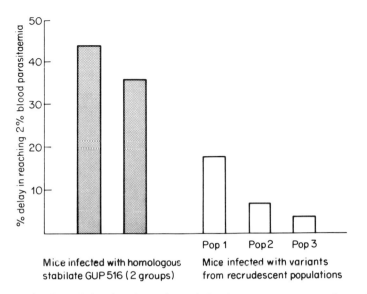

Fig. 4.6 Antigenic variation in *Plasmodium chabaudi*. Immune serum against stabilate GUP516 was injected into mice infected with this stabilate or with 3 stabilates derived from recrudescent populations appearing 31 to 33 days after initial infection with GUP516. The effect of the serum was measured by the length of time taken for the recipient mice to reach a 2% blood parasitaemia, and is expressed in terms of the percentage delay relative to controls. Activity against the homologous variant GUP516 resulted in delays of 2 to 4 days. (Data from McLean *et al.*, 1982, *Experimental Parasitology*, **54**, 296.)

lymphocytes. Such a mitogen, released *in vivo*, could lead to the polyclonal activation described above, although it is not clear precisely how this might lead to suppression of other responses. Suppression of antibody or plaque-forming responses has been demonstrated using both thymus-dependent and thymus-independent antigens (Fig. 4.7). The degree of suppression recorded varies between different model systems depending upon the severity and chronicity of infection. Delayed type hypersensitivity responses may also be suppressed in experimental infections. Both macrophages and non-specific T suppressor cells have been implicated in immune depression and it is possible that there may also be release of soluble factors from parasites which influence target cells directly. In general, immune suppression of responses to unrelated antigens co-exists with continuing responses to the parasite itself. However it has been shown that infections of mice with the erythrocytic stages of *P. berghei* prevents the induction of protection by vaccination with homologous sporozoites. Infection in both man and experimental animals produces profound changes in lymphoid organ structural organization and in populations of circulating cells. These changes may disrupt normal immune function and thus contribute to a generalized depression of responsiveness.

4.2 *Leishmania* and Leishmaniasis

All species of *Leishmania* are parasitic in cells of the mononuclear phagocytic series, cells with a primary function of phagocytosis and destruction of invading organisms and other foreign bodies. This seemingly paradoxical choice of host cell is shared with many bacterial pathogens and with a limited number of other protozoa

48

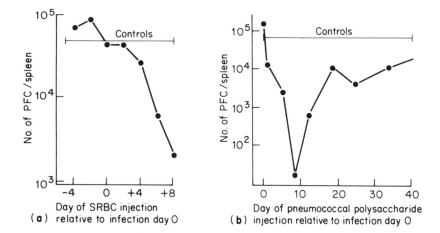

Fig. 4.7 Depression of immune responses in malaria infections. (a) Response to sheep red blood cells (SRBC) in mice infected with *P. berghei*. (b) Response to Type III pneumococcal polysaccharide in mice infected with *P. yoelii yoelii*. SRBC is a thymus-dependent antigen, pneumococcal polysaccharide is thymus independent. Response measured by counting number of direct plaque forming cells/spleen on day 5(A) or day 4(B). ((a) Redrawn from Liew *et al.*, 1979, *Immunology*, **37**, 35; (b) from McBride *et al.*, 1977, *Immunology*, **32**, 635.)

such as *Trypanosoma cruzi* and *Toxoplasma gondii*. All are capable of prolonged survival and reproduction within the macrophage and exhibit a variety of survival strategies. There are several species of *Leishmania* which can parasitize man and they give rise to a variety of diseases. The best known of these are Kala azar, a predominantly visceral form caused by *L. donovani*, Oriental Sore, a cutaneous lesion caused by *L. tropica*, and Espundia, a mucocutaneous infection caused by *L. brasiliensis*. The pathological manifestations of infection show wide variation, similar in many respects to the spectrum of disease conditions found in leprosy and likewise associated with the immunological state of the patient. This complexity is further compounded by the existence of numerous sub-species of *Leishmania* organisms.

The life cycles of all leishmanias follow a consistent pattern, and all use blood-feeding sand flies, species of phlebotomines, as vectors (Fig. 4.8). In all cases infections can be transmitted to man from a variety of animal reservoir hosts. Infection commences when promastigote forms are injected as the fly feeds. The promastigotes enter macrophages, transform into amastigotes and commence repeated binary fission; when infected cells burst, amastigotes are released and invade other macrophages. In *L. tropica* and *L. brasiliensis* infection remains localized within the skin and superficial tissues; in *L. donovani* infection spreads from the infected site to invade visceral organs. Flies become infected when they take up infected macrophages. The amastigotes are released in the insect's intestine, transform into promastigotes, undergo division and then move anteriorly into the proboscis.

In a typical form, *L. tropica* infection gives rise to ulcerative sores on the skin at the site of the sand-fly bite. Initially there is an infiltration of phagocytes in which amastigotes multiply; later lymphocytes accumulate and eventually the lesion resolves and heals. Infections with *L. brasiliensis* metastasize to the mucous membranes of the nose and mouth, eroding the cartilage and causing disfiguration. In

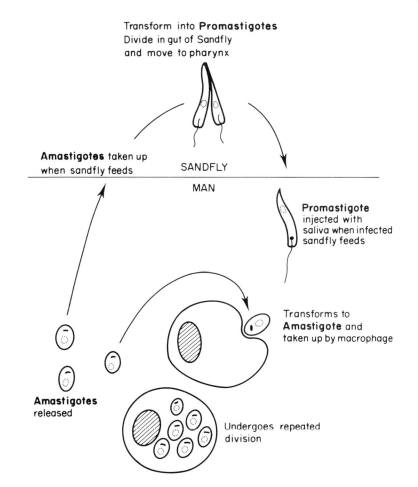

Transform into **Promastigotes**
Divide in gut of Sandfly
and move to pharynx

Amastigotes taken up
when sandfly feeds

SANDFLY

MAN

Promastigote
injected with
saliva when infected
sandfly feeds

Transforms to
Amastigote and
taken up by macrophage

Amastigotes
released

Undergoes repeated
division

Fig. 4.8 Life cycle of *Leishmania* in sandfly and man.

visceral leishmaniasis parasites spread from the site of infection and can be found almost all over the body. Parasite reproduction and cellular infiltrations lead to the characteristic enlargement of spleen and liver. A variety of other pathological changes may occur, including anaemia, haemorrhage, intestinal ulceration and damage to the heart.

4.2.1 Immunity to Leishmaniasis

It is difficult to make any generalized statements about immunity in the human leishmaniases, because there are so many exceptional circumstances to be considered. In simple forms *L. tropica* gives rise to infections that resolve spontaneously and leave the host with a strong immunity to re-infection, but this species is also associated with conditions (e.g. diffuse cutaneous leishmaniasis) where healing does not occur. Infections with *L. donovani* are progressive and usually fatal if not cured; after cure there is immunity to re-infection. The mucocutaneous leishmaniases, typified by *L. brasiliensis*, are often progressive and non-healing, but recovery can occur, with strong immunity to re-infection. In almost all cases immunity shows a rigid species and sub-species specificity.

Infection elicits strong cellular responses, measurable by delayed-type hypersensitivity reactions (DTH), and a rather variable antibody response. There is some correlation between DTH and ability to develop immunity, in that cell-mediated responses are reduced or absent in non-healing forms of the disease, and in these forms (the 'anergic' leishmaniases) there is normally a heavy parasitic load. Kala azar is characterized by a marked IgM and IgG hypergammaglobulinaemia, which probably reflects a massive polyclonal activation of B lymphocytes. Antibodies with parasite specificity are also produced, but these seem to play no role in host protection.

It is clear that the key to understanding the immunobiology of leishmanial infections lies in the relationship of the parasites to the host macrophages in which they live. A great deal of information relevant to this point has been obtained from *in vitro* studies and work with animal models, particularly in mice and Guinea pigs, in which infection can easily be initiated by direct injection of amastigotes (Table 4.4).

Table 4.4   Major laboratory models for immunological studies of leishmaniasis.

Host	Leishmania spp.	Disease
Mouse	L. mexicana	
	L. tropica	Cutaneous leishmaniasis
Guinea pig	L. enrietti	
Mouse	L. donovani	
		Visceral leishmaniasis
Hamster	L. donovani	

In Vitro *Studies*

The initial binding of parasites to the macrophage cell membrane is independent of Fc receptors and may not involve C3b receptors. It is possible that other glycoprotein or glycolipid molecules and receptors are involved and that their interaction leads to internalization by the conventional 'zipper mechanism' (Fig. 4.9). Certainly uptake can be blocked by inhibition of glycolysis in the host cell or by treatment with cytochalasin B. When completely internalized the parasite lies in a vacuole – the parasitophorous vacuole (Plate 4.5) – and is surrounded, more or less tightly, by host membrane. Lysosomal fusion with the vacuole occurs normally, but the amastigotes survive in the phagolysosome, even though lysosomal enzymes are present. (In this repect the survival strategy of *Leishmania* differs from those of *Toxoplasma*, which prevents lysosomal fusion from taking place, and *Trypanosoma cruzi*, which escapes from the vacuole into the cytoplasm.) Untransformed promastigotes cannot survive after phagocytosis and are destroyed.

The ability of amastigotes to survive and reproduce in what should be a hostile environment is not fully understood. The amastigote surface may be refractory to enzyme activity, or the amastigote may release factors which inhibit enzymes. It is known that parasite uptake by normal macrophages does not trigger the respiratory burst that ususally accompanies phagocytosis. As a result the parasites are not exposed to the oxygen metabolites (singlet oxygen, hydrogen peroxide, superoxide) that form an efficient antimicrobial defence. When macrophages are activated they

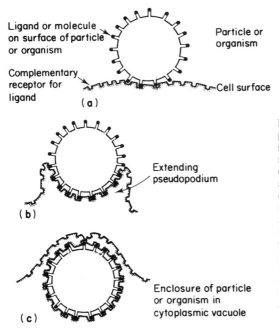

Ligand or molecule on surface of particle or organism

Particle or organism

Complementary receptor for ligand

Cell surface

(a)

Extending pseudopodium

(b)

Enclosure of particle or organism in cytoplasmic vacuole

(c)

Fig. 4.9 Interactions between particle or organism and host cell membrane which result in attachment (a) and then phagocytosis (b, c). Attachment may be achieved through a number of well-defined ligand-receptor interactions, including Ig and Fc receptors, C3b and C3b receptors as well as undefined interactions between surface sugars or glycoproteins and their complementary receptors. Internalization is normally an active, energy-dependent process. (Based upon Silverstein, 1977, *American Journal of Tropical Medicine and Hygiene*, **26**, 161.)

do produce these metabolites and amastigotes may then be killed. (Here again *T. gondii* shows a different strategy, surviving even when the respiratory burst is triggered, by virtue of its production of the enzymes superoxide dismutase and catalase which inactivate oxygen metabolites.)

Macrophage activation can be brought about in several ways, e.g. by injection of bacterial products and other materials, by exposure to infection, and by the action of lymphokines released from T lymphocytes. A variety of *in vitro* and *in vivo* studies have shown that activation is associated with parasite destruction. Thus, mice injected with BCG or with glucan are effectively protected against infection with *L. donovani* and *L. tropica.* Mouse macrophages exposed to supernatants from cultures of Con A stimulated spleen cells will kill *L. donovani* and *L. enrietti in vitro*. These demonstrations raise the question as to why leishmanial infections are often chronic and poorly controlled. Some answers have been obtained from studies of infections with *L. enrietti* in Guinea pigs and with *L. tropica* and *L. donovani* in mice.

In Vivo *Studies*

Infection with *L. enrietti* produces lesions akin to human Oriental Sore. Immunity develops with the resolution of the ulcer and the host is then strongly resistant to re-infection. DTH reactions to leishmanial antigen correlate with the existence of the immune state and there is also some evidence for formation of protective antibody. Transfer of immune serum can give some resistance to challenge, possibly by interfering with initial invasion of macrophages. When immunity is impaired by experimental manipulation of the host, or when very large numbers of parasites are injected (10^7–10^8 amastigotes), self-healing is not seen, chronic ulceration results and DTH reactions are lost. Although these observations provide a basis for studying the pathology and immunology of established non-healing infections they are essentially artificial. A more satisfactory model for the spectra of pathological and

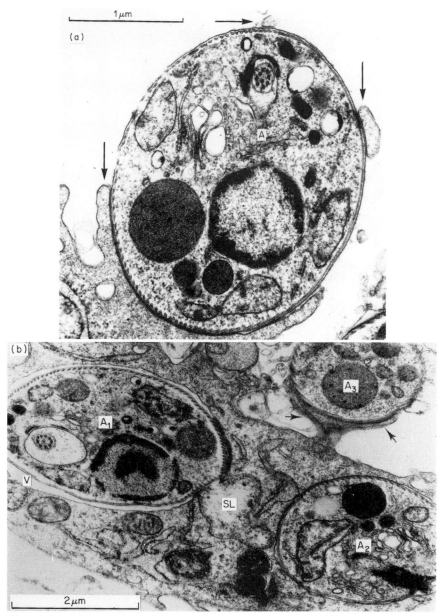

Plate 4.5 Uptake of *Leishmania* amastigotes by macrophages. (**a**) amastigote (A) being enveloped by macrophage pseudopodia (arrowed). (**b**) two amastigotes (A_1, A_2) within a macrophage 30 minutes after infection and a third (A_3) being enveloped by pseudopodia (arrowed). The intracellular parasites lie within membrane-bound parasitophorous vacuoles (V). A secondary lysosome (SL) is seen fusing with the vacuole and releasing contents. (Photographs from (a) Bray & Alexander (1983). In: *Leishmaniasis*, eds Killick-Kendrick & Peters, Academic Press, and (b) Blackwell & Alexander (1983). In: *Symposium on the Macrophage* ed. Willmott, *Trans. Roy. Soc. trop. Med. Hyg.* 77, 636. By permission of the authors and publishers.)

immunological responsiveness seen in human populations is provided by the use of mouse strains of defined genetic status, in which marked differences in susceptibility to *Leishmania* infections exist without prior manipulation.

L. donovani The existence of well-defined differences in response to infection was demonstrated in a panel of some 20 strains of mice. Two distinct patterns were apparent, resistant (R) and acutely susceptible (S) strains. In R mice there was very little replication in the liver; in S mice replication was unchecked and the animals became massively infected (Fig. 4.10). The difference between the most resistant and

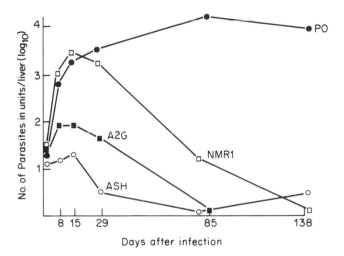

Fig. 4.10 Development of infections with *Leishmania donovani* in four strains of mice. (Redrawn from Bradley & Kirkley, 1977, *Clinical and experimental Immunology*, **30**, 130.)

most susceptible strains was such that there was a 1000-fold difference in liver parasite burdens within one month. S strains were further divisible into those capable of a later response which limited and then reduced infection and those incapable of this control. The basic distinction between R and S strains is apparent well before the intervention of immunity and reflects an innate difference in the ability of macrophages to support parasite development. In the first two weeks, replication in R mice is less than 8-fold; in S mice it is 80- to 100-fold. This innate difference is determined by a single gene, designated *Lsh*, which has been mapped to chromosome 1. The distinction between S strains in their capacity to control infections immunologically is dependent upon T cell-mediated responses and is regulated by genes linked to the H–2 (MHC) complex as well as by other genes. Resistance determined by *Lsh* is inherited as a dominant characteristic (Fig. 4.11A); resistance determined by H–2–linked genes is inherited as a recessive characteristic (Fig. 4.11B).

There is strong evidence that the gene *Lsh* is identical with the genes *Ity* and *Bcg* which determine susceptibility and resistance to two other intra-macrophage pathogens, namely *Salmonella typhimurium* and *Mycobacterium bovis* (BCG). It is logical therefore to assume that there is a common innate property of macrophages which determines their ability to support or resist the intracellular replication of these organisms. At present it is not known what this property is. It does not influence the initial process of entry into the macrophage, but differences between parasite development in R and S cells become apparent within a few days afterwards. The

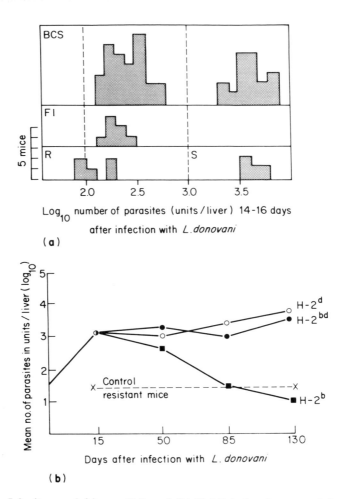

Fig. 4.11 Inheritance of (a) non H–2, and (b) H–2-linked resistance to infection with *Leishmania donovani* in mice. (a) Shows parasite liver burdens in mice derived by crossing resistant (R) and susceptible (S) strains (F₁) and by backcrossing F₁ to S parents (BCS). (b) Shows course of infection in H–2^d, H–2^b and hybrid H–2^{db} mice of the C57 BL/10 Sc Sn background. In (a) resistance is inherited as a dominant character, in (b) susceptibility is dominant. (Data from Bradley, 1974, *Nature*, **250**, 353; Blackwell *et al.*, 1980, *Nature*, **283**, 72.)

expression of the genetic control exercised by the H–2–linked genes is likewise unknown, although presumably it is reflected in the ability of macrophages to respond to lymphokines from sensitized T cells.

L. tropica   Clear-cut genetically-determined variation is also evident in infections of mouse strains with *L. tropica*. In highly resistant strains (NZB), infection does not establish at all; in resistant strains (C57BL), there is development of the characteristic skin ulcer, which then resolves; in susceptible strains (BALB/c) the lesion does not heal and visceral metastasis leads eventually to the death of the host. This stage of pathological manifestation reflects that known to occur in human infections with this species. The genetic control of susceptiblity and resistance to *L. tropica* is quite distinct from that of *L. donovani* and strains of mice may show quite opposite phenotypes when infected with the two species. Nevertheless, as in *L. donovani*, there appears to be a separate control of innate and acquired resistance, the latter again being a T-cell dependent phenomenon, antibody playing no major role. Athymic nude mice are highly susceptible to *L. tropica* but can be effectively protected by prior transfer of small numbers of Lyt 1^+ T cells from syngeneic donors. The level of resistance to *L. tropica* is primarily determined by a gene located on Chromosome 8; H–2–linked genes have a smaller influence than they do in *L. donovani*, although their influence can be critical. For example, whereas BALB/c mice (H2^d) acquire massive infections and die, BALB/K congenic mice (H2^k) eventually recover and survive.

Expression of genetic control is through macrophages and this can be shown directly by the behaviour of these cells when infected *in vitro* (Fig. 4.12) as well as by the course of infection in irradiated and bone marrow-reconstituted mice (Fig. 4.13). As with *L. donovani* the 'unsuitability' of resistant macrophages is not manifest at the stage of initial entry into the cell, but becomes apparent within a few days. The resistant phenotype is also associated with a qualitatively greater response to lymphokines, there being a good correlation between patterns of *in vivo* response status and *in vitro* macrophage response.

An important aspect of these genetic studies with *L. tropica* is the insight they have given into the relationship between extreme susceptibility (as shown by BALB/c mice) and immunosuppression. The failure of these mice to cure the infection is due to the selective induction of T suppressor cells. Deletion of this population of lymphocytes by treatment with irradiation, or cytotoxic drugs, allows recovery to occur. Elegant *in vitro* studies using a particular population of macrophage-type cells, the adherent fraction of skin cells, has shown that parasite growth is most rapid in a subset of small cells that can be isolated by virtue of their slow sedimentation. Infected cells from this population failed to present antigen adequately to immune lymphocytes, although uninfected cells functioned normally in this respect if pulsed with a parasite-antigen preparation, i.e. antigen handling was normal in uninfected cells of this subset. Infected cells also failed to immunize populations of naive lymphocytes, instead they selectively induced *Lyt* 2^+ T suppressor cells which were capable of interfering with sensitization of lymphocytes by skin adherent cells of resistant phenotype mice.

These results lead to the conclusion that the genetic defect in susceptible mice is reflected in an excessive antigen load in certain subsets of macrophages. It is also known that heavily-infected macrophages express reduced levels of self Ia antigens at their surfaces. The combination of high antigen concentration with reduced Ia expression specifically facilitates the induction of suppressor cells in lymphocyte populations.

How generally applicable this situation is, and to what extent it provides a model for the non-healing leishmaniases has yet to be determined. Certainly these infections appear to be correlated with immune suppression, but many other immunological factors may contribute to non-healing, including tolerance, blocking of effector function by immune complexes; non-immunological factors may also be involved. Nevertheless, in providing a conceptual framework, work with mouse models has proved particularly valuable. It has also shown the complexity of the interactions between host and parasite and how, in evolution there must have been a subtle interplay between the genotypes of both species for the chronic disease state to emerge.

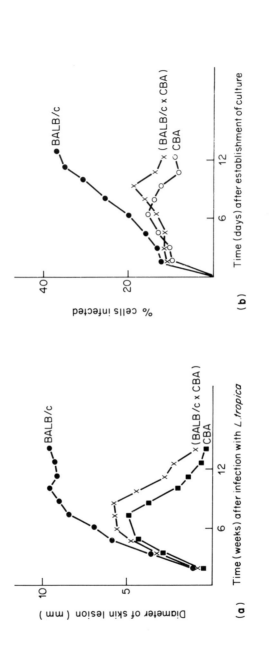

Fig. 4.12 Genetic control of immunity to *Leishmania tropica* in mice. (a) Growth of skin lesion in BALB/c, CBA and (BALB/c × CBA) F₁ mice after infection with 2 × 10⁷ organisms. (b) Time course of *in vitro* infection of skin adherent cells taken from the same strains of mice. (Redrawn from Gorczynski & MacRae, 1982, *Cellular Immunology*, **67**, 74.)

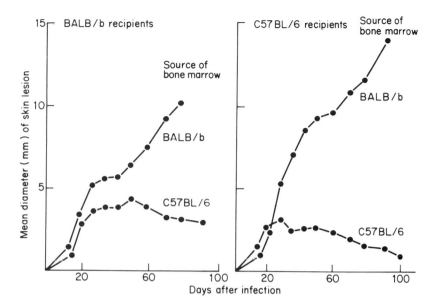

Fig. 4.13 Genetic control of immunity to *Leishmania tropica* in mice. Growth of skin lesion in radiation chimaeras after infection with 2×10^7 parasites. Chimaeras prepared by irradiating mice at 800 rads and injecting 5×10^6 syngeneic or H–2 compatible bone marrow. (Redrawn from Howard *et al.*, 1980, *Nature*, **288**, 161.)

5
African Trypanosomes
Antigenic Variation

5.1 Trypanosomiasis
5.2 Antigenic Variation
5.3 Mechanisms of Protective Immunity
5.4 Immune Suppression by Trypanosomes

Although the parasites discussed in the previous chapter are primarily intracellular organisms, they necessarily spend short periods outside the host cell. At these times they are demonstrably vulnerable to immunological attack. The African trypanosomes (genus *Trypanosoma*, section Salivaria) are the most important protozoa that live as extracellular parasites throughout the entire life cycle. Their long-term survival in this potentially hostile environment is primarily attributable to their ability to undergo antigenic variation, and thus keep one step ahead of the host's immune response. Our knowledge of this phenomenon represents, to date, one of the most completely understood of all parasite survival strategies.

Trypanosomes are flagellate protozoa, with a structural organization that is comparatively simple, even when examined under the electron-microscope. The life cycle typically includes a phase spent in the bloodstream and tissue fluids of a mammalian host, during which there is multiplication by binary fission, and a phase spent in the body of a vector arthropod (Fig. 5.1). For the majority of clinically and economically important species the arthropod concerned is a tsetse fly and the parasite undergoes major morphological and biochemical changes in this host, as well as repeated division. The parasites are taken up by the fly when it feeds on the blood of the mammalian host. Blood stream forms (trypomastigotes) are characteristically long and slender (Plate 5.1), with the kinetoplast situated posterior to the nucleus. The long, tubular mitochondrion is non-functional, the citric acid cycle and cytochrome system are absent and respiration occurs by glycolysis. A proportion of trypomastigotes are shorter, stumpy forms, and in these there is partial redevelopment of mitochondrial function. Only stumpy forms survive uptake by the tsetse fly. In the midgut the mitochondrion is functional and there is reappearance of the Krebs cycle and the cytochrome electron transport system. After extensive multiplication the midgut forms migrate anteriorly, between the peritrophic membrane and the gut wall and enter the salivary glands. There they differentiate, first into the epimastigote (anterior kinetoplast) and then, after further division, into the infective metacyclic form. Transmission is achieved when the infected tsetse next feeds, the metacyclics being introduced directly into the host with the saliva. (Experimental infections can be initiated directly by syringe passage of bloodstream forms.)

Tsetse flies occur only in a zone of equatorial Africa – the tsetse belt – and the requirement for cyclical development in this host restricts most trypanosome

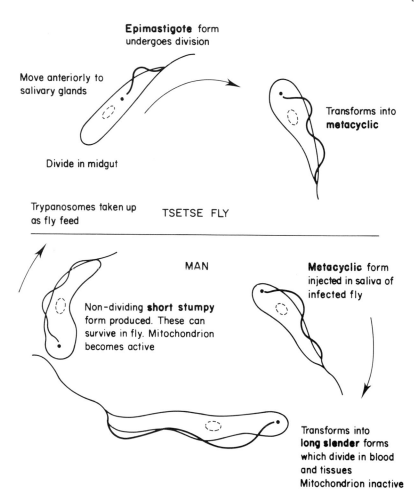

Epimastigote form
undergoes division

Move anteriorly to
salivary glands

Transforms into
metacyclic

Divide in midgut

Trypanosomes taken up
as fly feed

TSETSE FLY

MAN

Metacyclic form
injected in saliva of
infected fly

Non-dividing short stumpy
form produced. These can
survive in fly. Mitochondrion
becomes active

Transforms into
long slender forms
which divide in blood
and tissues
Mitochondrion inactive

Fig. 5.1 Life cycle of *Trypanosoma* in tsetse fly and man.

infections to this continent. However, direct transmission via the mouthparts of other biting flies is possible. In some species the requirement for cyclical development has been lost; transmission is therefore purely mechanical and can be achieved by a variety of blood-feeding flies and even by vampire bats. Such species, e.g. *T. evansi* and *T. equinum*, can survive outside the tsetse belt. In *T. equiperdum* transmission is achieved without the intervention of a vector and occurs venereally in equine hosts.

5.1 Trypanosomiasis

African trypanosomes are widespread in game animals, where they appear not to be unduly pathogenic. Trypanosomiasis as a recognizable and serious disease occurs in man, where it is caused by *T. brucei rhodesiense* and *T.b. gambiense*, and in domestic stock, where it is caused by several species, including *T.b. brucei*, *T. con-*

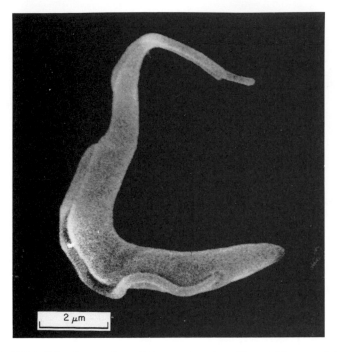

Plate 5.1 SEM of bloodstream form of *Trypanosoma brucei brucei*. (Photograph by courtesy of L. Tetley and Prof. K. Vickerman.)

golense and *T. vivax*. The only major differences between the sub-species of *T. brucei* appear to be infectivity for man and the nature of the disease caused by the two human parasites. Infections are associated with fever, anaemia, inflammation of lymph nodes, loss of weight and the lethargic condition from which the popular name of sleeping sickness is derived. Although trypanosomes appear initially in the blood they also move into the extravascular spaces of deeper tissues and frequently invade the central nervous system. It has been suggested that these tissue infections form a reservoir of dividing stages from which the blood infection is maintained.

Untreated infections are normally fatal, the time to death varying considerably. In man *T.b. gambiense* gives rise to a chronic infection, whereas infections with *T.b. rhodesiense* follow an acute course. There is no doubt that trypanosomiasis has a profound impact upon human development in Africa, not only through its direct effects in terms of human disease, but also indirectly through bovine infections, which prevent the utilization of grasslands for cattle farming. An estimated 35 million people and 25 million cattle are at risk from infection, and some 3 million cattle die annually from the disease.

5.2 Antigenic Variation

A characteristic feature of chronic trypanosome infections in man and animals is the occurrence of regular fluctuations in the numbers of parasites present in the blood (Fig. 5.2). This phenomenon has been recognized for very many years, and as long ago as 1907 it was suggested that each fall in the parasite population was brought about by the action of host antibodies. The subsequent rise in numbers was

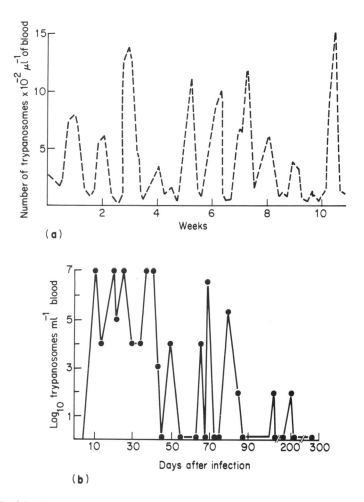

Fig. 5.2 (a) Fluctuations in numbers of trypanosomes in the blood of a sleeping sickness patient. (Redrawn from Ross & Thompson, 1910, *Proceedings of the Royal Society of London B*, **82**, 411.) (b) Fluctuations in the numbers of *Trypanosoma congolense* in the blood of a Zebu cow. (Redrawn from Murray *et al.*, 1980, *World Animal Review*, **32**, 9.)

interpreted as proliferation of parasites which differed antigenically from their predecessors. Contemporary research has shown this to be a remarkably accurate interpretation and there is now abundant evidence for sequential antigenic variation in the majority of salivarian trypanosomes. Variation does not appear to occur in stercorarian trypanosomes such as *T. cruzi*, which employ other strategies for survival (see p. 50). Most of our present data about antigenic variation comes from work using *T.b. brucei*, a species which can be maintained without difficulty in convenient laboratory hosts. There is good evidence, however, from work with human trypanosomes and with *T. congolense* and *T. equiperdum*, that what is true of *T.b. brucei* is likely to be substantially true for the other salivarian species.

Antigenic variation can be detected directly by a variety of immunological techniques, using antibodies with specificity for particular variant antigenic types (VATs). These techniques include immunofluorescence, agglutination, neutralization of infectivity and complement-mediated lysis. In each case, trypanosomes carrying an unrelated VAT are unaffected, thus validating the interpretation of fluctuating parasitaemias described above. In the host, binding of antibodies to trypanosomes would result in their removal from the bloodstream. Those that were unaffected would multiply to provide the next peak of parasitaemia, before again being destroyed by antibodies with specificity for their particular VAT.

5.2.1   The Surface Glycoprotein Coat

The ability of antibodies to agglutinate or lyse trypanosomes implies the existence of antigens upon the surface of the parasite. Such antigens can be visualized by EM techniques using ferritin-labelled antisera which bind to the surface of trypanosomes carrying the homologous VAT (Plate 5.2). Unlike most cell membranes, those of bloodstream trypanosomes are covered by a prominent surface coat, some 12–15 nm thick. Biochemical analyses have shown that the major, probably the sole component of this coat is a single species of glycoprotein molecule of approximately 60 kD to 65 kD molecular weight. The molecules are thought to be arranged as a monolayer and collectively constitute about 10% of the dry weight of the organism (Fig. 5.3).

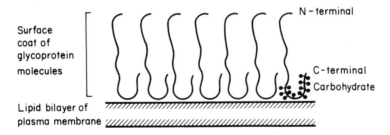

Fig. 5.3 Relationship of glycoprotein surface coat to plasma membrane of trypanosome. (Redrawn from Cross & Johnson, 1976, In *Biochemistry of Parasites and Host–Parasite Relationships* (ed. H. Van den Bossche), Elsevier, p. 413.)

Compared with erythrocytes, which have a comparable surface area, trypanosomes have a such greater density (at least 10×) of glycoprotein molecules at their cell surface, and clearly this glycoprotein layer must perform an important biological function. Much circumstantial evidence pointed to the glycoproteins as the trypanosome surface antigen, and this has now been proved conclusively. Thus, when trypansomes differentiate in the tsetse fly, the surface coat is lost, as it is when the protozoa are maintained under certain culture conditions (Plate 5.2). In both cases, loss of the coat is correlated with loss of antigenicity. Conversely, the redevelopment of the coat by the metacyclic stage is associated with reappearance of antigenicity. This replaceable coat can be thought of as an adaptation for survival in the bloodstream of the mammalian host and protection against the host's immune response naturally comes to mind. Certainly the glycoprotein coat appears to be inpenetrable to a variety of macromolecules, and stages without the coat do not survive in the mammalian host. Nevertheless the glycoproteins themselves can be the focus for immune responses with the potential to destroy the organisms which bear them. Direct evidence for this comes from experiments which have shown that, in the mouse, injection of as little as 3 μg of purified glycoprotein confers complete

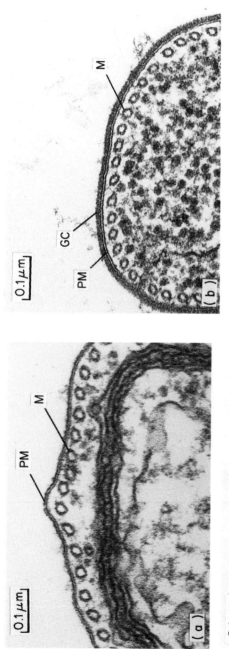

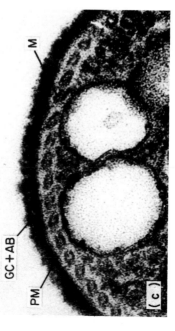

Plate 5.2 The glycoprotein surface coat of *Trypanosoma brucei brucei*. (a) TEM of 26°C culture form in which the glycoprotein coat has been lost. (b) TEM of bloodstream form showing the thick glycoprotein coat covering the plasma membrane. (c) TEM of bloodstream form exposed firstly to a mouse monoclonal antibody with specificity for the variant antigen in the glycoprotein coat, and then to a rabbit anti-mouse antibody conjugated with horse radish peroxidase. GC = glycoprotein coat, GC + AB = glycoprotein coat with antibody, M = microtubule, PM = plasma membrane. (Photographs by courtesy of L. Tetley and Prof. K. Vickerman.)

protection against infection with trypanosomes carrying the homologous antigen. This protection is highly specific and has no effect upon parasites of a different VAT. Herein lies a paradox. Immunity can be elicited by antigens present in the surface coat, and is highly specific. Cross-reacting antigens, known to be common to many variant populations, seem to elicit immune responses with little or no protective capacity. Why then do trypanosomes cover themselves with highly immunogenic material, responses to which bring about their destruction? It may well be that the glycoprotein coat is a necessary requirement for survival in the physiological environment of the bloodstream, but an equally attractive suggestion is that, by provoking effective mechanisms of host control, yet possessing the capacity to undergo antigenic variation, trypanosomes optimize their survival. Uncontrolled growth of infections, as is seen with 'virulent' strains or as occurs in immuno-compromised animals, is rapidly fatal to the host. Fluctuating parasitaemias, on the other hand, may persist for prolonged periods, giving a greater opportunity for transmission to a new host.

5.2.2   Variation in Surface Glycoproteins

It is possible, using manipulative techniques and short-term infections in rodents, to clone large numbers of identical trypanosomes carrying a single VAT and thus to obtain sufficient material to analyse surface glycoproteins in detail (Fig. 5.4).

Single trypanosomes are isolated by microscopic examination of drop preparations and injected into lethally irradiated hosts. After 3 to 4 days parasites are removed from the first host, and injected into a second irradiated host. The process is repeated until sufficient numbers of trypanosomes are available. The parasites are separated from the blood by centrifugation and passage through an anion-exchange column. Samples of the populations can be cryopreserved to form stabilates from which new infections of the same VAT can be derived when required. When the surface coats of trypanosomes cloned from representatives of several different VATs are studied and compared, it is found that in each case, purification of their glycoproteins gives a single and homogeneous molecular species. These are comparable between VATs in molecular weight but vary extensively in composition. The antigenic variation that gives rise to distinct VATs is therefore brought about by expression in the surface coat of variant specific glycoproteins (VSGs).

A great deal is now known of the detailed structure and organization of VSGs. The molecules appear not to penetrate the lipid bilayer of the plasma membrane to any extent, being anchored by a hydrophobic peptide extension. They are mobile upon the surface, as can be shown by the phenomenon of capping in the presence of specific antibody. The carbohydrate components of the molecule (galactose, glucose, mannose and glucosamine) are located basally, close to the membrane attachment and probably contribute little to the serological distinctiveness of the VSG. Indeed, cross-reactivity between VSGs of different clones has been located to the C-terminal carbohydrates. Variation between VSGs does occur in the amount and proportion of the different sugars but is most marked in the amino acid sequences of the polypeptide chain. In five VATs studied, for example, there was no homology at all between the N-terminal sequences (Fig. 5.5) and immense variation in the C-terminal sequences.

5.2.3   Expression of VSGs during Infection

One of the major questions that arose from the formal demonstration of antigenic variation was the nature of the mechanisms, in both host and parasite, which were responsible for the appearance of VSGs during the course of a trypanosome

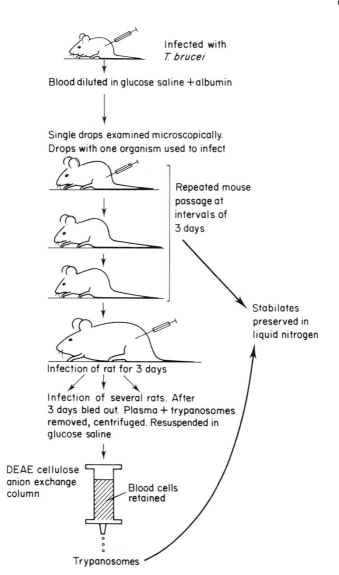

Infected with
T. brucei

Blood diluted in glucose saline + albumin

Single drops examined microscopically.
Drops with one organism used to infect

Repeated mouse
passage at
intervals of
3 days

Stabilates
preserved in
liquid nitrogen

Infection of rat for 3 days

Infection of several rats. After
3 days bled out. Plasma + trypanosomes
removed, centrifuged. Resuspended in
glucose saline

DEAE cellulose
anion exchange
column

Blood cells
retained

Trypanosomes

Fig. 5.4 Techniques used for obtaining large numbers of cloned trypanosomes for biochemical and immunological studies. (Based on Cross, 1975, *Parasitology*, **71**, 393.)

infection. Progress in this area has been greatly facilitated by the development of investigative approaches using the techniques of modern immunology and molecular biology. An early suggestion was that antigenic variation was induced in a population by the development of antibodies against the surface glycoproteins. Although it is difficult to exclude this completely, there is much experimental evidence to show that VSGs appear in populations established in irradiated hosts (i.e. hosts unable to respond immunologically) and in populations passaged between hosts at intervals

Variant antigen			5					10					15					20
1	Thr Asn Asn His Gly Leu Lys Leu Gln Lys Ala Glu Ala Lle Cys Lys Met Cys Lys Glu
2	Ala Lys Glu Ala Leu Glu Tyr Lys Thr Trp Thr Asn His Cys Gly Leu Ala Ala Thr Leu
3	Thr Asp Lys Gly Ala Lle Lys Phe Glu Thr Trp Glu Pro Leu Gln Leu Leu Thr Gln Asp
4	Ala Glu Ala Lys Ser Asp Thr Ala Ser Gly Ser Val Asn Ser Pro Gln Thr Glu Ala Thr

Fig. 5.5 N-terminal amino acid sequences of four variant antigens isolated from one clone of *Trypanosoma brucei* (only the first 20 amino acids are shown). (Data from Cross, 1977, *American Journal of Tropical Medicine and Hygiene*, **26**, 240.)

shorter than that required for the expression of antibody responses. More convincing evidence that antibody is not essential has come from studies involving *in vitro* culture. It is now possible to maintain bloodstream forms for long periods *in vitro* and antigenic variation has been recorded under these conditions. It therefore appears that the major role of antibody *in vivo* is to eliminate trypanosomes carrying the predominant VSG, allowing multiplication of parasites with different antigens. This see-saw relationship between host and parasite gives rise to the characteristic fluctuations in parasitaemia. Detailed studies on infections initiated with cloned parasites, using sensitive and highly specific serological techniques, have shown that although the population present during the rising phase of a peak consists predominantly of one VAT (the homotype), minor VATs (heterotypes) are also present. Once the homotype population crashes, any of the heterotypes may become the homotype of the next peak (Fig. 5.6).

The rate at which antigenic variation occurs in infections established with cloned parasites (1 in $10^4/10^5$ organisms) is such that genetic mutation could be the underlying mechanism. However, there is now much circumstantial evidence that this is not the case. One of the strongest arguments against mutation as the major cause of variation came from early studies on the sequences in which VSGs were expressed during infection. These showed that, using defined infections of *T.b. brucei*, certain VSGs were consistently expressed early in infection and were followed by a regular and reasonably predictable sequence of predominant VSGs thereafter, at least until the later stages of a chronic infection. When particular VATs are cloned and one clone used to establish infections in different individual animals, the sequence of VSGs produced in the hosts is similar. Each clone seems therefore to have a characteristic repertoire of VSGs (collectively referred to as a serodeme), presumably determined by its genotype; some of the VSGs may be shared with other serodemes. The total number of VSGs may be very large, for example more than 100 have been recorded in infections with *T. equiperdum*.

The theoretical and practical importance of predictable patterns of VSG expression has prompted many detailed studies. The most recent suggest that the predictability is not as clear-cut as originally assumed. Earlier studies used agglutination or lysis of populations by antibody in order to determine VSG, whereas the development of monospecific antisera derived from immunization with specific VSGs, allows the use of immunofluorescence to type individual organisms. Nevertheless, it is still evident that there is a statistically definable order of priority in which VSGs are expressed, but the precise order may differ according to the parent VAT. Within particular clones particular VSGs, the predominant types, have relatively high probabilities of expression. Differential growth rates, and therefore

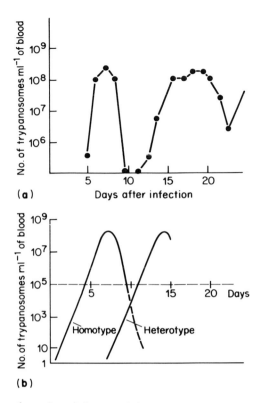

Fig. 5.6 (a) Course of parasitaemia in mouse infected with single trypanosome on day 0. First peak is distinct, due to growth of predominant VAT (homotype). Relapse peaks less distinct, because of overlapping growth of heterotypes. (b) Theoretical picture showing growth of homotype and relapse arising from growth of heterotype. Only one heterotype is shown, in practice several might be present simultaneously. One heterotype becomes the predominant VAT of the relapse peak that follows remission of the original homotype. 10^5 represents the detectable level of patent parasitaemias. (Both redrawn from Vickerman, 1978, *Nature*, **273**, 613.)

competition between VATs, play an important part in determining which types are likely to emerge as the major VATs, particularly during the early phases of infections.

The existence of predictability in sequences of variation and the demonstration of VSG repertoires argue against mutation as an underlying mechanism. So also does the fact that, when populations derived from cloned parasites are cyclically passaged through tsetse flies, they appear to revert to a basic antigen type from which the sequence of antigenic change recommences after infection of the mammalian host. This latter observation is of course of major importance when potential means of immunological control are being considered. If it is true that, in each serodeme, there is reversion to a single antigenic type during development of metacyclic forms in the tsetse fly, then it follows that the first population peak in fly-transmitted infections should always show this VAT and it should therefore be possible to vaccinate against infection. Even though populations of tsetse flies in endemic areas might transmit metacyclic trypanosomes derived from several serodemes, restrictions of antigenic variability to that seen between basic VATs makes a very much easier target for vaccination than the enormous range of VSGs that each serodeme is capable of producing. Unfortunately it does not now appear that the metacyclics of a given serodeme all carry the same VSG, even though a majority may do so. Analysis of metacyclic forms originating from a single VSG-defined population has shown heterogeneity in immunofluorescent staining and susceptibility to lysis with monospecific antisera. For example, at least four VSGs, and probably more, were present in the metacyclics produced in flies fed upon mice infected with VSG defined population of the AnTAR 1 serodeme, and all of these were different from

Table 5.1   Antigenic variation in metacyclic trypanosome (*T.b. brucei*) populations from tsetse flies. Flies were fed on mice infected with particular VATs from the AnTAR 1 serodeme and the antigenic type of the resultant metacyclic forms determined using antisera against specific VATs. (Data from Hajduk *et al.*, 1981, *Parasitology*, **83**, 595.)

		% metacyclics labelled using immunofluorescent antisera against:			
VAT homotype ingested	% heterotypes ingested tryps	Ingested homotype		Metacyclic VATs	
			AnTat 1.6	AnTat 1.30	AnTat 1.45
AnTat 1.8	0.5	0.0	4.0	20.5	10.0
AnTat 1.14	20.6	0.0	6.0	22.5	4.7
AnTat 1.18	3.9	0.0	0.0	22.5	2.7
AnTat 1.19	0.3	0.0	9.0	18.2	3.0
AnTat 1.21	0.2	0.0	5.5	19.1	4.9

the VSG of the homotype ingested (Table 5.1). When mice were infected with parasites from these flies the metacyclic VSGs were the first to be identified in the blood stream forms, the VSG of the ingested homotype appearing later. This variability at source is further compounded by the rapidity of variation occurring immediately after infection. As many as 19 distinct VSGs have been demonstrated in the population present during the first peak of parasitaemia arising from a fly-transmitted infection (Table 5.2).

5.2.4   Genetic Control of VSG Expression

If mututation is not the major cause of the antigenic variation seen both in the fly and in the bloodstream of the mammalian host, then variation must arise from the expression of alternative genes, there being a non-random switching between genes to provide the degree of predictability observed in VSG succession. Some progress has been made in elucidating the mechanisms of genetic control through which this switching occurs, but little is known of the way in which the phenotype of the surface coat is changed on the individual trypanosome. It is clear that individual organisms must have the ability to change, but whether there is a stage at which two VSGs are present simultaneously, or whether one coat is removed by capping and another put on is unknown. Simultaneous fluorescence with antisera directed against two distinct surface antigens has been described in individuals from a population grown *in vitro*, and although this may be an abnormal situation it does provide a means of studying this question.

Analyses of the nuclear DNA of trypanosomes, in relation to antigenic variation, has been carried out using cDNA prepared from the mRNA coding for a specific

Table 5.2 Appearance of VATs in bloodstream trypanosomes (*T. b. brucei*) following infection of mice by tsetse flies fed on donors harbouring a VAT defined population. (Data from Hajduk & Vickerman, 1981, *Parasitology*, **83**, 609.)

VAT homotype ingested by fly	Days after fly bite	Fluorescence obtained with monospecific antisera against AnTat VATs																							
		1	2	3	4	5	6*	7	8	9	10	11	12	13	14	15	16	17	18	19	20	21	22	30*	45*
AnTat 1.8	3	−	−	−	−	−	−	−	−	−	−	−	−	−	−	−	−	−	−	−	−	−	−	+	+
	5	−	+	+	+	−	+	+	+	+	+	+	+	−	+	+	+	+	+	−	−	−	−	+	+
	7	−	+	+	+	−	+	+	+	+	+	+	−	−	+	+	−	+	+	−	−	−	−	−	−
	9	−	+	−	+	−	+	+	+	−	−	−	−	−	−	+	+	−	+	+	−	−	−	−	−
AnTat 1.18	3	−	−	−	−	−	+	+	+	−	−	−	−	−	+	+	+	−	−	−	+	−	−	+	+
	5	−	+	+	−	+	+	+	−	+	+	+	+	+	+	+	+	+	+	+	+	+	−	−	+
	7	−	−	+	+	+	+	+	−	+	−	+	+	−	−	+	+	−	+	+	+	+	−	−	−
	9	−	+	+	+	−	+	+	+	−	−	−	−	−	+	+	+	+	+	+	−	−	−	−	−

* VATs identified within the metacyclic population (see Table 5.1).

VSG of the AnTAR 1 serodeme. (In any one cloned population the only VSG mRNA detectable is that of the VSG present at the cell surface.) In preparations of homologous genomic DNA, hybridization with the cDNA probe revealed several incomplete and two complete copies of the gene sequence, one of 6.4 kilobases (kb) and one of 2 kb. The latter was present only from DNA from trypanosomes expressing the specific glycoprotein, being absent in other variants of the same serodeme. The 6.4 kb copy, however, was present in these variants and it is therefore considered to be the basic copy of the gene, acting as the template from which the expression linked 2 kb copy is generated. This conclusion is further supported by the fact that the 2 kb copy was absent in culture-induced procyclic forms which lack the surface coat and corresponding VSG.

It therefore appears that, in a given serodeme, all the trypanosomes carry all the genes coding for the VSGs in the repertoire, but the expression of these genes is regulated at the transcriptional level. Expression involves duplication of the coding sequence and transposition of the copy to an expression site. The factors which initiate and control this process are unknown, but could include endogenous programming as well as exogenous triggering by a variety of environmental factors, of which antibody might be one in certain circumstances.

5.3   Mechanisms of Protective Immunity

As will be apparent from the above, the failure of hosts to control trypanosome infections results primarily from the phenomenon of antigenic variation and not from an inability to mount protective responses. The effectiveness of such responses can be seen when, under controlled conditions, immunity is stimulated by injection of purified VSG or by vaccination with irradiated organisms. Certain breeds of cattle appear able to develop some immunity in the field and this can be enhanced by judicious use of chemotherapy to abbreviate natural infections.

The mechanisms underlying protective responses can only be investigated in laboratory systems where immunizing procedures and challenge infections can be precisely regulated. In these models it is easy to demonstrate highly efficient anti-trypanosome responses mediated by antibodies directed against the surface antigens. For example, when a VSG-specific monoclonal antibody was injected into mice with a moderate parasitaemia of *T.b. brucei* (10^7 ml^{-1}) the parasites were cleared from the bloodstream within 20 minutes. Transfer of immunity can also be achieved using serum or B lymphocytes from infected animals. *In vitro* studies show that antibodies can lyse trypanosomes in the presence of complement, but complement is not necessary for the *in vivo* clearance of bloodstream forms. IgM antibodies seem to be the most effective in this clearance and this is borne out by the fact that thymus-deficient (nude) and thymus-deprived mice can control an initial parasitaemia as successfully as normal mice. It has been suggested that, in the mouse at least, control is achieved through IgM antibodies acting initially as trypano-agglutinins, agglutination itself being sufficient to cause lysis. Other studies using direct injection of trypanosomes labelled with an isotope of methionine, have shown that antibody-mediated clearance from the blood is brought about by phagocytosis in the liver (Fig. 5.7). Phagocytosis can be induced by passive transfer of small volumes of immune serum, or by prior incubation of parasites in serum, and is complement independent. Although no positive evidence was presented, it was concluded from this work that prior lysis of trypanosomes was not a necessary prerequisite for uptake by the liver.

Cell-mediated responses appear to play no major role in protective immunity, although they may contribute to the development of the 'chancre', a lesion which appears at the site of tsetse bites and which may localize and destroy some of the parasites.

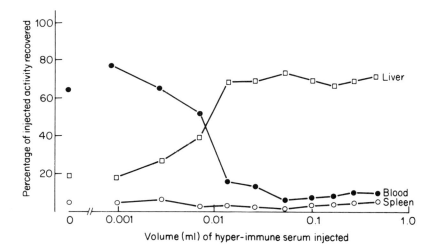

Fig. 5.7 Distribution of radio-labelled (^{75}Se) trypanosomes (*T.b. brucei*) 60 minutes after injection into mice passively immunized with various amounts of serum from rats immunized against the homologous parasite. (Redrawn from MacAskill *et al.*, 1980, *Immunology*, **40**, 629.)

5.4 Immune Suppression by Trypanosomes

Trypanosome infections give rise to pronounced suppression of immune responses in man, bovines and experimental animals. This suppression is operative against responses to a wide variety of heterologous antigens, including prophylactic vaccines, other infectious organisms and defined antigens such as sheep RBC. Paradoxically suppression is coincident with very substantial increases in circulating immunoglobulin, particularly IgM. Indeed IgM hypergammaglobulinaemia is, in endemic areas, diagnostic of trypanosomiasis.

The production of well-defined antibody responses to VSGs and the frequent antigenic variation in chronic, relapsing infections would be expected to lead to a large increase in circulating immunoglobulin. However, the level of this response in trypanosomiasis is such that only a proportion of the immunoglobulin is likely to be specific anti-trypanosome antibody, the remainder being immunoglobulin produced as a result of parasite-induced polyclonal activation of B cells. It is of course difficult to be sure that antibody is not specific for the parasite unless all antigen specificities can be tested, but support for the concept of a polyclonal activation comes from experimental studies with mice infected with *T.b. brucei*. Within one week of infection with 10^5 trypanosomes the spleen contained elevated numbers of IgM plaque-forming cells secreting antibodies against heterologous antigens such as sheep RBC, chicken gamma globulin, pneumococcal polysaccharide, and the hapten TNP (Fig. 5.8). Autoantibodies against single-stranded DNA, mouse RBC and thymocytes were also detected. The degree of polyclonal antibody synthesis was comparable in infected nude mice and infected normal mice, implying that the effect of the trypanosomes is independent of any positive or negative T cell-mediated effects upon the B cell population.

It is well established that polyclonal B-cell activators may suppress immune responses when given before injection of antigen and it has been suggested that an important element in the pronounced immunosuppression associated with trypanosomiasis (Fig. 5.9) is the mitogenic effect which trypanosomes have upon the cells of the host. One way in which this may lead to suppression could be exhaustion of antigen-specific B cells, leading to a loss of response to mitogens and antigens as

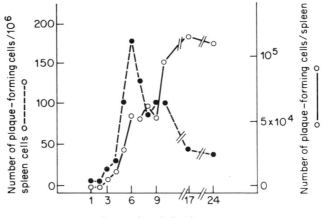

Fig. 5.8 Increase in number of B cells producing anti-TNP (trinitrophenyl) antibody after infection of mice with *T.b. brucei*. Number of cells measured by plaque forming assay. (Redrawn from Kobayakawa *et al.*, 1979, *Journal of Immunology*, **122**, 296.)

well as loss of immunological memory. The nature of the mitogen involved and the way in which it acts upon B cells are uncertain. Polyclonal activation and immune suppression can be induced *in vivo* by injection of irradiated trypanosomes or of membrane fractions of the parasites, but *in vitro* studies of this phenomenon using living trypanosomes have, in general, been unsatisfactory.

Polyclonal activation may certainly be a major factor in immune suppression, but it has been demonstrated repeatedly that infections also lead to the production of non-specific T cells and of suppressor or inhibitory macrophages; general lymphocyte dysfunction is also marked. T suppressor cells appear early after experimental infection with *T.b. brucei*, within one week. Their effects upon *in vitro* responses of spleen cells to B cell mitogens such as LPS can be reversed by their removal from the cell population. Later on in infection removal of suppressor T cells does not reverse suppression, showing a more fundamental loss of activity in B cells. The suppressive effects associated with infection can be transferred to naive mice with peritoneal macrophages from infected donors or with macrophages that have phagocytosed irradiated trypanosomes. There is some evidence that the mitogenic and suppressive properties of trypanosome material are evident only after macrophage processing, and may arise from some fundamental alteration of the immunoregulatory functions of these cells.

A most important, and much debated point, is the effect that trypanosome-induced suppression has upon homologous immunity, i.e. upon responses to trypanosomes as such, and the effect to which it contributes towards the failure to control infection. Evidence on this point is conflicting. In mice infected with certain virulent serodemes of *T.b. brucei* the pattern of parasitaemia suggests a strong antibody-mediated control of the first peak but very little control of the second. With other serodemes there appears to be successively weaker control of subsequent peaks. One explanation for this observation could be that there is a depression in immune capacity, but another could be the emergence of a number of variants, each being partially but not completely controlled. When depression of immune capacity is achieved by treating infected mice with immunosuppressants there is a rapid and unrestricted rise in parasitaemia followed by death. However, in acute infections, the

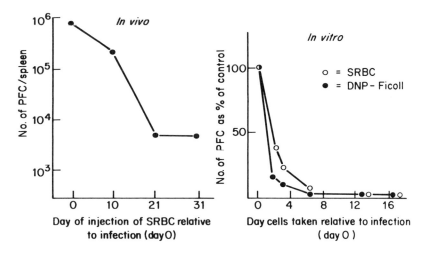

Fig. 5.9 Depression of immune responses in mice infected with *Trypanosoma brucei.* (**a**) *In vivo*: Mice infected with *T.b. brucei* were injected with sheep red blood cells (SRBC) at intervals after infection. Response was measured as the number of plaque-forming cells (PFC) 5 days after injection. (**b**) *In vitro*: Spleen cells were removed from mice at intervals after infection with *T.b. brucei* and immunized *in vitro* with SRBC or DNP–Ficoll. Response was measured as the number of PFC per culture of 10^7 cells. (**a**) Data from Hudson & Terry, 1979, *Parasite Immunology*, **1**, 317; (**b**) Redrawn from Eardley & Jayawardena, 1977, *Journal of Immunology*, **119**, 1029.)

failure to control parasitaemia arises not from depression of the level of response, but from the swamping of protective capacity by the sheer number of trypanosomes present. If numbers are reduced by chemotherapy the levels of antibody present are adequate to clear the bloodstream.

Experiments with *T.b. brucei* in mice have failed to show that infection with live organisms of one VAT can suppress immunity to another VAT generated by vaccination with irradiated organisms. In contrast, in cattle, it has been shown that after simultaneous infection with two different clones of *T.b. brucei* or of *T. congolense*, the variant specific antibody response to one clone was depressed whilst responses to the other were not. This depression was not seen if infection with the second clone was delayed for more than two days, suggesting a form of antigenic competition. A decisive factor determining depression of responses to VSGs in a chronic infection may therefore be the time at which new variants arise and the rate at which each population multiplies. Faster growing populations are more likely to exert a suppressive effect on other variants because they expose the host to a greater amount of antigen. However, it is also possible that their ability to multiply more rapidly may be a consequence rather than a cause of their immunosuppressive properties, i.e. they may depress homologous as well as heterologous responses.

The complexity of the immunological interactions between host and trypanosome and the antigenic variability inherent in the latter pose formidable problems for the development of pratical and effective methods of controlling trypanosomiasis by immunological means. Although a great deal is now understood about antigenicity in these organisms it has so far proved impossible to make use of this knowledge in effective control under field conditions. Trypanosomes continue to promote their own survival, not only by circumventing and depleting the hosts' immune response but also by outwitting the efforts of immunoparasitologists.

6

Schistosomes

Concomitant Immunity and Immunopathology

The immunobiology of infections with helminths differs in two important respects from that of infections with protozoa. Helminths are many times larger than protozoans and do not replicate within the vertebrate host. The difference in size restricts the ways in which hosts can mount effective immune responses and the lack of replication influences the survival strategies of both host and parasite. These points will be considered initially in the context of infections with schistosomes.

Schistosomes are platyhelminth (flatworm) parasites which live as adults in the blood vessels of their mammalian and bird hosts. The majority of parasitic flatworms are hermaphrodite, but schistosomes are not. Their generic name, which means 'split-body', describes the appearance presented by the individual males and females, which live as permanent couples, the larger, fatter male carrying the female in a longitudinal groove. The life cycle is indirect and involves a molluscan intermediate host (Fig. 6.1). Eggs are released from the body of the final host via faeces or urine, depending upon the species of schistosome. They are mature when released and, on contact with fresh water, hatch to liberate the first larval stage, the miracidium. This small, ciliated organism has limited powers of survival and must come into contact with the correct species of aquatic snail if the cycle is to continue. When contact is made, the miracidium penetrates into the snail, losing the ciliated epidermis as it does so, and transforms into the sporocyst. The sporocyst has a syncytial, cytoplasmic outer surface and, having no digestive system, absorbs nutrients directly across this layer. Within its body, permanently embryonic cells divide and differentiate to form a second generation of sporocysts. In these, similar cells divide and differentiate to form the next larval stage, the cercaria. By this process of asexual division the schistosome can greatly increase its reproductive potential. In *S. mansoni*, a species which infects man, it has been calculated that one miracidium is capable of producing 200 000 cercariae. The cercaria is the stage infective to the final host. It leaves the snail and becomes temporarily free-living. The larva shows characteristic behaviour patterns, hanging from the surface film of the body of water into which it has been released, detaching, sinking, then swimming upwards again. By so doing it may increase the chances of coming into contact with a suitable host.

Infection of the final host occurs by direct penetration of the skin. The cercaria first attaches to the epidermis, sheds its tail and then, by a combination of vigorous movement and enzyme secretion, penetrates through the epidermis, crosses the

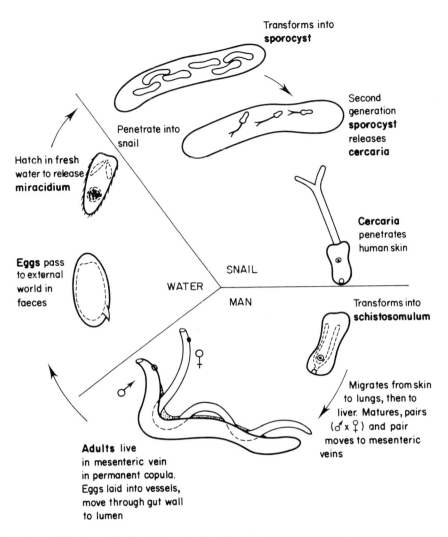

Transforms into
sporocyst

Penetrate into
snail

Second
generation
sporocyst
releases
cercaria

Hatch in fresh
water to release
miracidium

Cercaria
penetrates
human skin

Eggs pass
to external
world in
faeces

SNAIL

WATER

MAN

Transforms into
schistosomulum

Migrates from skin
to lungs, then to
liver. Matures, pairs
(♂ x ♀) and pair
moves to mesenteric
veins

Adults live
in mesenteric vein
in permanent copula.
Eggs laid into vessels,
move through gut wall
to lumen

Fig. 6.1 Life cycle of schistosome in snail and man (based on *S. mansoni*).

basement membrane and enters the dermis. On penetration the cercaria undergoes profound changes in the structure and physiological properties of the surface layer, the tegument. Whereas the cercarial surface is bounded by a trilaminate plasma membrane, bearing a thick glycocalyx, the tegument of the succeeding stage, the schistosomulum, develops a multilaminate plasma membrane, the glycocalyx is lost and the larvae becomes unable to survive in water (Fig. 6.2). After a period of time the schistosomulum migrates via the blood stream to the lungs and from there to the liver. Following growth and maturation in this organ, the adult worms pair and move into the veins of the mesenteries or into those surrounding the urinary bladder. The complete cycle, from egg release to full sexual maturity may take several weeks.

Once mature the worms survive for a considerable time, possibly as long as five or

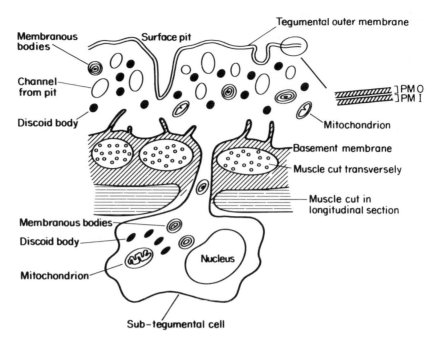

Fig. 6.2 Diagrammatic representation of the tegument of an adult schistosome seen at the ultrastructural level. PMI, PMO = Inner and outer plasma membranes. (Redrawn from McLaren, 1980, *Schistosoma mansoni: The Parasite Surface in Relation to Host Immunity*, Wiley, London.)

six years, during which they release a very large number of eggs (*S. mansoni* 300 per day; *S. japonicum* 3000 per day). Eggs are laid by the females into small diameter vessels and become trapped by the elasticity of the vessel wall. Their passage from the vessel, across the tissues to the lumen of the intestine or bladder is dependent upon enzymes released from the miracidia, which develop precociously within the eggs. As will be seen later, it is this phase of the life cycle that is responsible for the severe pathology associated with schistosomiasis.

6.1 Schistosomiasis

Infections with schistosomes are widely distributed in tropical and sub-tropical regions, their distribution being limited by the climatic conditions appropriate for the survival of the snail hosts. Human schistosomiasis, which affects some 300×10^6 people, is caused primarily by three species, *S. mansoni* (Africa, Central and South America), *S. japonicum* (Asia), and *S. haematobium* (Africa). In the first two species the adult worms live in the mesenteric veins of the intestine; *S. haematobium* inhabits the plexus of veins around the bladder. Several species, notably *S. bovis* and *S. mattei*, cause disease and severe economic loss in cattle and sheep. In all hosts schistosomiasis is a chronic and insidious disease, producing long-term, debilitating pathology.

6.2   Immune Responses

As may be expected from the fact that the host is parasitized for long periods by relatively large and reproductively prolific parasites, infection is associated with a wide variety of immune responses. Initial penetration of the skin produces little reaction, but in repeated infections there may be local hypersensitivity responses. (In man such responses are much more pronounced after infection by the cercariae of avian schistosomes. These are unable to develop further, die in the skin and give rise to a violent dermatitis-swimmers' itch.) Early development is sometimes associated with acute allergic reactions, but often the first responses that become evident are those associated with the production of eggs. The constant release of potent immunogens from the eggs produces a strong cell-mediated immunity and this leads to pronounced immunopathological changes (see p. 89). The adult worms are themselves not directly pathogenic, but they are strongly immunogenic. Antigenic material is released from the tegument, from the intestine, and is also released during metabolism. A variety of antibody responses is made to these antigens, including marked reaginic responses.

6.3   Protective Immunity

Despite the abundant evidence for immunological responsiveness to infection there is, in man, very little clear-cut evidence for acquired immunity and infections persist for very long periods. Circumstantial evidence for resistance has been drawn from the survival of populations in areas with high transmission rates and from the fact that infection levels, measured by egg output, plateau after the second decade of life (Fig. 6.3). Nevertheless it has to be borne in mind that many other factors, including changes in degree of water contact, may contribute to such overall patterns of infection and survival.

In animal models there is clear evidence of immunity, the precise form of immunity depending upon the species of host used. With *S. mansoni*, for example, rhesus

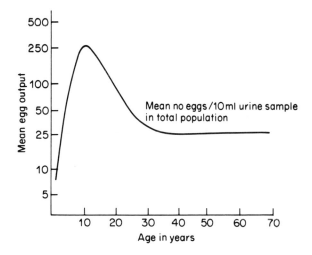

Fig. 6.3   Prevalence of infection with *Schistosoma haematobium* in a population living in an endemic area. (Data from Bradley & McCullough, 1973, *Transactions of the Royal Society for Tropical Medicine and Hygiene,* **67**, 491.)

monkeys express very substantial immunity on re-infection, but primary infections survive for many months; baboons show less resistance to challenge infections. In the rat, primary infections are themselves terminated by immunity and there is strong resistance to re-infection. Mice on the other hand are closer to the rhesus monkey in their overall responses to infection.

Some of the most important experimental studies of the mechanisms underlying immunity to schistosomes were carried out by Smithers and Terry during the 1960s. The results they obtained have exerted a very significant influence upon subsequent approaches to this question. In summary their work with *S. mansoni* showed that:

(*a*) Rhesus monkeys were able to destroy the majority of worms developing from a challenge infection, but did not eliminate the adults that had established from the initial infection.

(*b*) Immunity to infection could be stimulated by exposure to large numbers of attenuated (irradiated) cercariae or by transplantation of adult worms directly into the vascular system.

(*c*) Immunity to re-infection appeared to act against the larval stages. Because this immunity could be stimulated by adult worms, the two stages must express common antigens, yet the adults were unaffected by responses that destroyed the larvae.

In 1969 Smithers and Terry proposed the term *concomitant immunity* to describe this paradoxical situation in rhesus monkeys. This term was taken from tumour immunology, where it was used to describe the fact that animals bearing certain primary tumours were able to destroy new tumours of the same kind but were unable to control the initial tumour. It is now recognized that concomitant immunity to schistosomes exists in other hosts and subsequent work has elucidated much about the ways in which adult worms evade the immune response and in which developing larvae are killed. These two aspects will be discussed separately.

6.3.1   Evasion of Immunity by Adult worms

At the time that the concept of concomitant immunity in schistosomiasis was put forward it was already known that, in homogenates of adult worms, there were antigens which were indistinguishable from those of the host used for the infection. It was realized that the existence of such common antigens would help to reduce antigenic disparity between host and parasite and thereby decrease the impact of immune responses. Smithers and Terry provided direct evidence to support this proposition by carrying out the experiments shown in Fig. 6.4. Immunization against mouse antigens was achieved by injecting monkeys with homogenized liver and spleen cells, with RBC or with serum proteins. When worms were transferred from monkey donors survival was essentially similar whether the recipient had been immunized against mouse antigens or not. 'Mouse' worms survived after transfer into normal monkeys but required about 6 weeks to regain pre-transfer levels of egg output. In monkeys immunized against mouse antigens the majority of 'mouse' worms died within 25 hours and all were dead after 44 hours.

It was also shown in these experiments that the immunity operative against 'mouse' worms in anti-mouse monkeys was transferable with serum, that immune damage occurred at the surface of the worm, and the the susceptibility of 'mouse' worms to the immune environment of anti-mouse monkeys was lost if they were first passaged through a normal monkey. After one week the 'mouse' worms become monkey adapted and were not killed after transfer into immunized recipients.

It follows from these results that worms acquire from their hosts molecules, called by Smithers and Terry 'host antigens', and have the ability to turn over these molecules at a relatively rapid rate, i.e. they can be replaced within one week. The

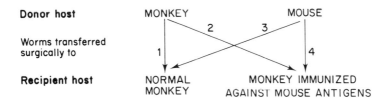

Donor host MONKEY   MOUSE

Worms transferred
surgically to

Recipient host NORMAL   MONKEY IMMUNIZED
                    MONKEY   AGAINST MOUSE ANTIGENS

Outcome of transfer:

1. MONKEY ⟶ NORMAL MONKEY. Worms survived, no interruption
   of egg laying.

2. MONKEY ⟶ ANTI-MOUSE MONKEY. Worms survived, no interruption
   of egg laying.

3. MOUSE ⟶ NORMAL MONKEY. Worms survived, egg laying interrupted
   for 5-6 weeks.

4. MOUSE ⟶ ANTI-MOUSE MONKEY. All worms killed within 44 hours.

Fig. 6.4 Protocol of experiments used to demonstrate presence of host antigens on the tegument of adult *Schistosoma mansoni*. (Data from Smithers *et al.*, 1969, *Proceedings of the Royal Society B*, **171**, 483.)

host antigens are present at the surface of the worm, as can be seen by their interaction with antibodies in the immunized recipient. From the fact that adult worms do stimulate specific and potentially destructive immune responses, but are not themselves affected, it may be inferred that host antigens play a protective role, disguising the surface of the worm so that it is seen as self and thus preventing interaction with host immune mediators.

This view of the way in which adult schistosomes evade the immune response has been somewhat modified over recent years, but still remains an acceptable explanation. Support for the concept of acquisition of host antigens was provided by *in vitro* experimentation using the early schistosomula stages. It was readily shown that larvae cultured in medium containing human RBC would acquire on their tegumental surface the glycolipid antigens of the major blood groups A and B. If larvae were subsequently transplanted into monkeys immunized against these blood group antigens they were rapidly killed (Table 6.1). Glycoprotein antigens of the M, N, S and Duffy blood groups were not acquired. More recent work has shown that schistosomula can acquire a variety of host molecules, including histocompatibility antigens, immunoglobulins and skin intercellular-substance antigens. In no case, however, is it understood how such molecules are acquired. There is, in addition, good evidence that schistosomes can actively synthesize molecules which cross react with host antigens. The sum total of these molecules on the tegument must play a major role in protecting worms from immune attack, but this disguise is not the only protective strategy used by the parasite. The surface of the tegument is constantly replaced by membrane formed in deeper-lying tissues and this turnover appears to be accelerated when the surface is subjected to antibody plus complement-mediated attack. In addition, there is increasing evidence that in development the tegument of

Table 6.1 Acquisition of human red blood cell (RBC) antigens by schistosomula of *Schistosoma mansoni* during *in vitro* culture, measured by their susceptibility to anti-RBC antibodies after transfer into monkeys immunized with human RBC in Freund's Complete Adjuvant (FCA). (Data from Clegg *et al.*, 1971, *Nature*, **232**, 653.)

Type of RBC included in in vitro *culture medium*	Immunization of recipient monkey	% of transferred larvae recovered as adults
Monkey	FCA	67
Monkey	None	79
Human (A.B.Rh−)	FCA	73
Human (A.B.Rh−)	None	45
Monkey	Human RBC in FCA	103
Monkey	Human RBC in FCA	96
Human (A.B.Rh−)	Human RBC in FCA	3
Human (A.B.Rh−)	Human RBC in FCA	5

the schistosomulum undergoes a series of changes, the net effect of which is to render the worm relatively insusceptible to immune-mediated damage. (This particular point is elaborated further in the following section.) However, this latter strategy seems less relevant to the survival of the adults than it is for earlier stages. This was neatly demonstrated by the experiment shown in Fig. 6.5. Taking advantage of the fact that host antigens are bound to the tegument, lung-stage and adult worms from mice were incubated in neat inactivated anti-mouse RBC antisera and then exposed to rat eosinophils. Cell adherence occurred with both stages, and degranulation was also demonstrated. Despite this, damage and death was only evident with the adult worms; lung worms were unaffected. Neither stage bound antibodies directed against schistosome antigens. This property was shown only in 3 hour skin-penetrated schistosomula. Thus the 'disguise' of the adults is a necessary protection, as their tegument is clearly susceptible to cell-mediated damage if the disguise is by-passed.

6.3.2   Effector Mechanisms

Although in general adult worms appear well protected, they can be affected by immune responses generated by infection. In rhesus monkeys, for example, the egg output of worms maturing from a primary infection with *S. mansoni* reaches a peak after 8 to 12 weeks. It then falls rapidly to a much lower level, which may be maintained for a very long period. In rats, the majority of adult *S. mansoni* are eliminated between the 4th and 8th week. However, despite this evidence for effective anti-adult immunity, it seems that the most important targets for effector mechanisms are the early schistosomula which develop from challenge infections. The nature of the effectors and their interaction with the larvae have been intensively studied *in vitro* as well as by manipulative *in vivo* experiments. Both approaches have been facilitated by the development of techniques for the production of schistosomula directly from cercaria, either by penetration through a skin membrane (skin-transformed schistosomula) or after mechanical agitation (mechanically-transformed schistosomula) – see Fig. 6.6. The schistosomula can be maintained for long periods in relatively simple media, they will also establish infections in experimental hosts after intravenous injection.

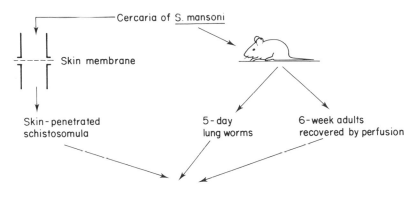

Incubated in microtitre plates (37°C, 5% CO_2) together with test serum, or test serum and eosinophils taken from rats.

Results

1. BINDING OF ANTIBODY − DETECTED BY IMMUNOFLUORESCENCE WITH FITC-LABELLED GOAT ANTI-RAT IgG.

	Fluorescence		
Test serum	Skin s/somula	Lung worms	Adult
normal rat (NRS)	−ve	−ve	−ve
immune rat (anti-schistosome) (IRS)	++++	−ve	$\mp$
rat anti-mouse RBC (RAM)	+	++++	++++

2. EOSINOPHIL-MEDIATED CYTOTOXICITY IN HEAT-INACTIVATED SERA

	% Dead worms after 48 H		
Test serum	Skin s/somula	Lung worms	Adult
NRS	<5%	<5%	<5%
IRS	20%	5%	<5%
RAM	<15%	5%	50%

Fig. 6.5 Protocol of experiment used to demonstrate binding of anti-parasite and anti-host antibody to developmental stages of *Schistosoma mansoni* in the mouse and the ability of antibody to mediate eosinophil killing. (Data taken from McLaren & Terry, 1982, *Parasite Immunology*, **4**, 129.)

6.3.3 *In Vitro* Studies

It is possible to test the ability of various effector mechanisms to damage and destroy schistosomula merely by adding components to *in vitro* cultures of the larvae. The viability of the worms can be assessed in a number of ways, by uptake or exclusion of vital dyes, by release of isotope markers, by changes in morphology or by ability to establish infections, and the detailed course of the interactions between effectors and parasite can be monitored biochemically or microscopically. A variety

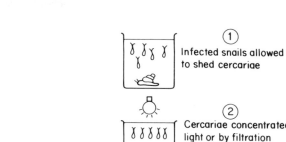

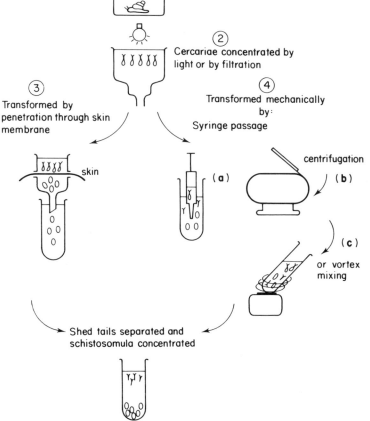

Fig. 6.6 Summary of techniques used to prepare schistosomula stages of schistosomes for experimental studies. (1) Infected snails are exposed to light to stimulate release of cercariae. (2) Cercariae are concentrated using filtration, or using their positive responses towards light. Two techniques may then be used. (3) Cercariae are allowed to penetrate a membrane prepared from rat skin and the schistosomula collected after penetration. (4) Cercariae are agitated mechanically by (a) repeated passage into and out of a syringe, (b) centrifugation, or (c) vortex mixing. The cercariae lose their tails and transform into schistosomula.

There are differences between schistosomula prepared by each technique, reflected most obviously in susceptibility to *in vitro* killing. Schistosomula may be cryopreserved after preparation.

of potential effectors have been examined, in a variety of host-parasite combinations. Those which have been shown to damage larvae are summarized in Table 6.2. As can be seen, almost all involve cooperative interactions between cells and antibodies. Only one system relies wholly on antibody alone. Complement-mediated lysis occurs in the presence of anti-worm IgG antibody (lethal antibody) taken from hyper-infected hosts. Such antibody is known to occur in man and many experimental hosts,

Table 6.2 Cells and antibodies known to be effective in the *in vitro* killing of schistosomula larvae. (From Capron *et al.*, 1982, *Immunological Reviews*, **61**, 41.)

Cell	Antibody isotype	Host species
Neutrophil	IgG	Rat
Eosinophil	IgG	Man
Eosinophil	IgG2a	Rat
Eosinophil	IgG	Mouse
Eosinophil	IgE	Rat
Macrophage	IgE	Rat
Monocyte	IgE	Man, Baboon

and can also be induced by vaccination with surface membrane fractions derived from adult worms. Despite the effectiveness of this mechanism *in vitro*, no effect is seen when the antibody is passively transferred into infected hosts and its biological significance remains uncertain.

The interaction of effector cells with larvae (Plate 6.1) occurs through membrane receptors for Fc or C3b, or after specific arming by antigen–antibody complexes. Eosinophils, neutrophils and macrophages can all function as effectors in such reactions. The former are probably the most efficient killer cells and may have the most important role *in vivo*.

6.3.4 Eosinophils

Eosinophils will adhere to schistosomula that have been coated with antibody through their receptors for the Fc portions of immunoglobulin molecules. Adherence also occurs through the membrane C3b receptor and, as the larval tegument activates complement by the alternate pathway, can take place in the absence of specific antibody. Killing appears most efficient in the presence of both antibody and complement although substantial killing will take when either is present alone (Fig. 6.7). This may reflect the greater number of C3 molecules bound to the larval surface after complement activation by the classical pathway, but the attraction of cells by chemotactic factors released during activation must also play a role. When all components are present simultaneously killing of schistosomula can exceed 80% within 3 hours.

Initial studies showed that eosinophil-mediated killing occurred in the presence of IgG antibodies and it was of interest that in the rat, the subclass involved was IgG2a, the isotype which also attaches to mast cells. These antibodies have specificity for antigens present on the worm's surface and can be absorbed with membrane fractions prepared from either larval or adult stages, i.e. there are identical, or cross-reacting, antigens in both stages. Immune complexes formed between IgG and antigens can also render eosinophils cytotoxic. More recently it has also been shown that eosinophil killing can be mediated through IgE antibodies, an entirely novel aspect of the functions of this isotype. An interesting observation is that in rat hosts, there is a switch between isotypes capable of mediating eosinophil killing during the course of infection. Before 6 weeks IgG antibodies are present, after this time IgE antibodies predominate.

Killing of schistosomula by eosinophils is enhanced in the presence of mast cells, and this enhancement is associated with the release by these cells of soluble mediators, now known to be the chemotactic tetrapeptides of ECF–A (the eosinophil chemotactic factor of anaphylaxis). The precise mechanism involved is uncertain, but

84

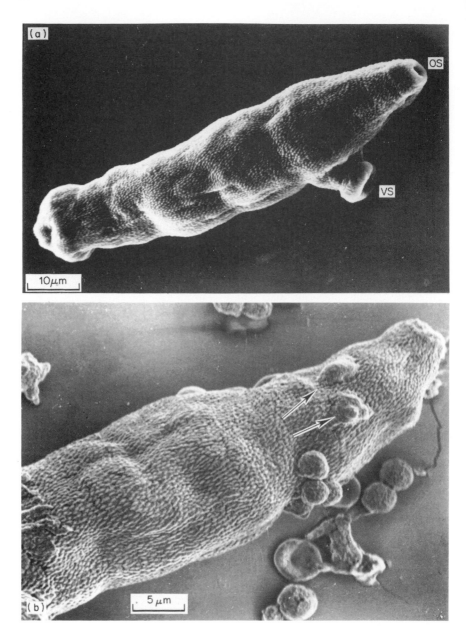

Plate 6.1 *In vitro* adherence of cells (eosinophils) to schistosomula larvae of *Schistosoma mansoni*. (a) Schistosomulum after preparation showing oral (OS) and ventral (VS) suckers and tegumental spines. (b) Schistosomulum after incubation with antibody and human eosinophils. Some of the cells are still rounded, others (arrowed) are flattened onto the tegument. (Photographs by courtesy of Drs A.M. Glauert and A.E. Butterworth.)

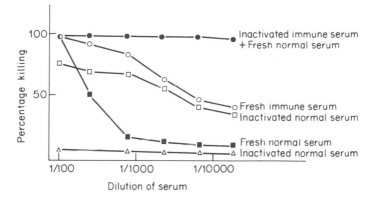

Fig. 6.7 Mediation of eosinophil cytotoxicity against schistosomula of *Schistosoma mansoni* by various rat sera. (Inactivated sera were heated at 56°C for 60 min to destroy complement.) (Redrawn from McLaren & Ramalho-Pinto, 1979, *Journal of Immunology*, **123**, 1431.)

it may well be correlated with the increase in receptor density that is known to occur when eosinophils are exposed to these mediators and thus reflect a more efficient adherence to the worm. Alternatively or additionally, as eosinophil peroxidases are known to bind to mast cell granules, and thereby acquire a greater bactericidal activity, there may be a more effective killing in the presence of mast cells.

After adherence to the larvae, eosinophils flatten out and make intimate contact with the worm's surface (Plate 6.2a). The secretion granules of the cell accumulate adjacent to the point of contact and fuse to form vacuoles (Plate 6.2b). Eventually the vacuoles fuse with the cell membrane and their contents are released onto the worm (Plate 6.2c). It is known that the secretion granules contain a variety of factors, including enzymes such as peroxidases and phospholipase B, which can damage the tegument of the parasite. They also contain large, characteristically-shaped crystalline bodies, which have as a major component a strongly basic protein. This major basic protein (MBP) is also released and exerts a potent destructive effect; *in vitro*, isolated MBP damaged larvae at concentrations as low as 2×10^{-5}M.

Damage occurs initially at the outer bilayer of the tegumental membrane, and then at the inner bilayer. These changes alter the permeability of the membranes and vacuolation occurs in the tegument itself. Eosinophils then actively invade the tegument and strip it away from the underlying musculature (Plate 6.2d).

6.3.5 Neutrophils

These cells, like eosinophils, can adhere to schistosomula through IgG Fc and C3b receptors. However, there are many differences in the kinetics of *in vitro* responses and in the effects of these cells upon the parasite. Adherence is less intimate than with eosinophils, and neutrophils readily detach. Recent observations have revealed that, under certain conditions, detachment results in part of the neutrophil membrane remaining behind as a 'footprint', i.e. the cell membrane becomes fused with parasite tegumental membrane. It has been suggested that the events leading to this fusion and detachment represent a protective strategy by the worm, preventing prolonged contact with potentially harmful effectors. Under optimal conditions, and with complement-mediated adherence, neutrophils readily kill worms; this killing is achieved by release of a variety of enzymes from the neutrophil granules and may also

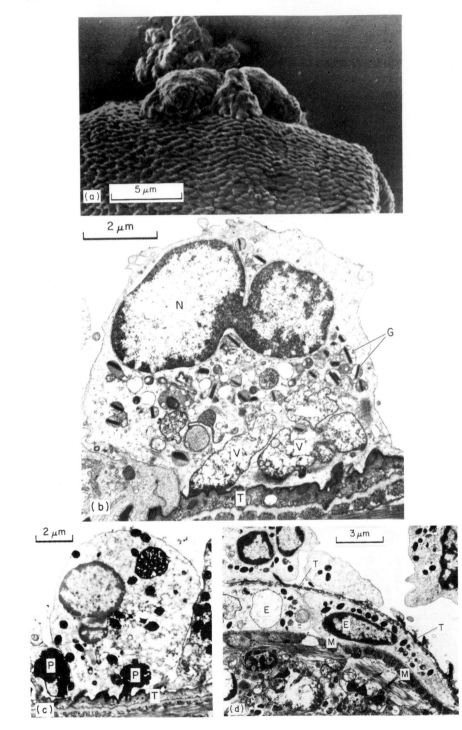

involve products of the respiratory burst. Unlike eosinophil damage, neutrophil-mediated damage appears first in the internal tissues of the worm. During the initial period the tegument remains apparently intact, although, as release of isotope markers shows, substantial permeability changes occur. Later, tegumental damage is evident, cells insert pseudopodia into the tegument and extensive areas disintegrate.

6.3.5 Macrophages

Macrophage-mediated killing of schistosomula appears to function through two distinct mechanisms. One is associated with macrophage activation and is therefore essentially non-specific in action, the other involves immune complexes between IgE and parasite antigen and therefore is induced specifically. In the latter the complexes attach to the macrophage through membrane receptors for IgE and thus arm and activate the macrophage rather than opsonize the parasite. IgG antibody seems to play no role in this particular system, indeed cleavage by parasite enzymes of anti-parasite IgG releases peptides that interfere with IgE-dependent macrophage cytotoxicity.

It is striking that neither natural killer cells nor cytotoxic T lymphocytes appear to be effective in anti-schistosomular killing even though both cell types function effectively in killing tumour cells, a partially analogous target. The failure of lymphocytes to kill schistosomula is more remarkable when it is considered that the parasites acquire host MHC antigens on their surfaces and therefore potentially have the necessary self and foreign stimuli to elicit cytotoxic responses.

6.3.7 Schistosomula as Targets for Effector Mechanisms

In vitro killing is effective only if the target schistosomula are young. After only a few days, their susceptibility is lost and effector mechanisms have little effect. This rapid acquisition of defences is of course essential to the survival of the parasite even during primary infections. Although antibodies are not present, the surface of the schistosomulum can activate complement via the alternative pathway and therefore can elicit C3b-mediated cell adherence. Loss of susceptibility is correlated with a loss of surface antigenicity, thus antibodies bind less well, and with a loss of ability to activate complement, but it is at the same time associated with a greater resistance to

---

Plate 6.2 Eosinophil-mediated cytotoxicity against schistosomula larvae of *Schistosoma mansoni*. (**a**) Eosinophils adhering to the tegument. (**b**) Close adherence of eosinophil and fusion of granules (G) to form vacuoles (V). N = nucleus of eosinophil, T = tegument. (**c**) Release of peroxidase-stained material (P) from vacuoles onto the tegument (T). (**d**) Destruction of tegument (T) by invading cells (E). M = muscle layer of schistosomulum. (a) by courtesy of Drs A.M. Glauert and A.E. Butterworth. (b) and (d) from McLaren *et al.*, 1978, *Parasitology*, **77**, 313. (c) from McLaren, 1980, *Schistosoma mansoni: The Parasite Surface in Relation to Host Immunity*, Research Studies Press, John Wiley. By permission of the authors and publishers.)

effector-mediated damage. This has been elegantly demonstrated by making older schistosomula artificially immunogenic (by linking haptens to their surface) and then exposing them to complement- and eosinophil-mediated attack (Table 6.3). The reasons for these changes in the larvae and their increased resistance are not fully understood. There is evidence that exposure to factors present in human sera triggers biochemical changes in the tegument, one result of which is uptake of neutral lipids. Such changes may lead to masking of antigenic sites and reduction in binding of complement. However there is also evidence for acquisition of resistance even when larvae are cultured in serum-free media.

Table 6.3   Resistance of lung-stage larvae of *Schistosoma mansoni* to antibody-mediated killing by eosinophils. Larvae were haptenated by coupling trinitrophenyl (TNP) to the tegumental surface, and incubated at 37°C *in vitro* with rabbit anti-TNP antisera and purified human eosinophils. (Data from Moser *et al.*, 1980, *Journal of experimental Medicine*, **152**, 41.)

Larvae	% of larvae with > 5 adherent eosinophils at 18h	% degranulated eosinophils on larvae at 18h	% larvae killed after 36h
3 hours-old skin stage	88.8	53.3	80.5
5 days-old lung stage	100.0	63.3	15.2

6.3.8   *In Vivo* Studies

In vitro experimentation has revealed a great deal about potential effector mechanisms, but it is obviously important to know which of these mechanisms function *in vivo* and to know the extent to which they contribute to overall resistance. It has been established from many experimental approaches that resistance is thymus dependent, but this dependency may operate at several levels, e.g. in antibody formation, in myeloid cell responses or in cell-mediated immunity. It has been possible to transfer immunity passively with serum (IgG) and recently this has also been achieved using monoclonal IgG antibodies known to be directed against tegumental antigens. It has also been shown that antibody is effective only if there is cooperation with cellular elements (Table 6.4). Rats treated with anti-μ chain antisera from birth, and thus incapable of forming immunoglobulins, show greatly reduced resistance, as do mice treated with antisera that eliminate eosinophils. Eosinophil involvement in worm destruction is deduced from histopathological studies of infections initiated by normal percutaneous infection as well as those initiated by intravenous injection of schistosomula. The latter technique enables detailed time-course studies to be made of responses to the larvae as they migrate through the lungs.

The manipulability of schistosome infections in laboratory hosts, and the ease with which hosts can be immunized by controlled infections or by vaccination procedures, makes it possible to identify the stages affected by resistance mechanisms. Direct worm recovery is possible from the skin, lung and mesenteric veins, and sites where worms have been trapped and destroyed (sites of attrition) can be identified histologically and by tracking isotopically-labelled worms. It is clear that there is

Table 6.4 Requirement for bone marrow-derived cells in expression of antibody mediated immunity against intravenously injected schistosomula of *Schistosoma mansoni*. (Data from Sher, 1977, *American Journal of Tropical Medicine and Hygiene*, **26**, 20.)

Group of mice	Mean number of larvae recovered from lungs after 5 days
1. Given normal rat serum	81
2. Given immune rat serum	39
3. Irradiated at 650 rads 13 days before immune serum	109
4. Irradiated at 650 rads and given bone marrow cells 13 days before immune serum	50

considerable variation between hosts in the sites at which challenge infections are affected by immunity. Variation also arises depending on the means used to stimulate immunity (i.e. infection or vaccination) and the route of challenge (i.e. at the same site as or different from the immunizing infection). In one set of experiments, in which animals were made immune by vaccination with attenuated larvae, it was found that the major site of attrition of *S. mansoni* in mice was the skin, in rats the lung and in guinea pigs the lung and liver. Attrition in the skin of mice has been demonstrated by many workers, but there is also evidence for a later effect upon worms, after they have left the lungs (Fig. 6.8). This effect is more pronounced in mice immunized by chronic infections than in those immunized by vaccination. It is possible that it is mediated by non-specific inflammatory effects associated with granuloma formation in the liver (see below), as worms at this age are not susceptible to antibody-mediated cytotoxicity, but another possibility is that the liver pathology associated with chronic infections results in young worms being diverted through porto-caval anastomoses, with the result that they are lost elsewhere. Some support from this idea is given by the quite different pattern of worm recoveries in vaccinated mice (Fig. 6.8) where the major loss of worms occurs well before the liver is reached.

6.4 Immunopathology

Schistosomiasis is one of several parasitic diseases in which the pathology associated with infection is caused not by the direct activities of the parasite, but by the immunological and inflammatory responses of the host. There are a number of well-defined immunopathological symptoms associated with infection, including the dermatitis that may follow cercarial penetration, the acute allergic phase caused by parasite migration through the lungs, the later phase (Katayama fever) seen in *S. japonicum* infections and immune-complex disease. The most intensively studied immuno-pathological reactions are those associated with chronic *S. mansoni* infections and which are responsible for the gross changes seen in the liver. The close similarity between schistosomiasis in man and that in mice has allowed the underlying causes of this pathology to be studied in great detail.

The intended fate of the eggs released from the female *S. mansoni* in the mesenteric vessels is their movement into the tissues and lumen of the intestine and their ultimate release from the host in faecal material. Many eggs, however, do not remain localized in the blood vessels around the intestine, but are swept away by the blood. They enter the hepatic portal vein, pass into the liver and then become

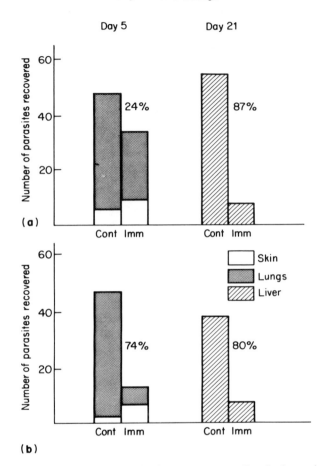

Fig. 6.8 Site of attrition of an infection of *Schistosoma mansoni* in mice immunized, (a) by infection with 20 cercariae 4 months previously, and (b) by infection with 400 cercariae irradiated at 20 k rad. The figures above the bars represent the percentage reduction in recovery compared with the controls. Day 5 worms recovered from excised and chopped lungs; day 21 worms recovered by liver perfusion. (Redrawn from Smithers & Miller, 1980, *American Journal of Tropical Medicine and Hygiene*, **29**, 832.)

trapped in pre-sinusoidal venules. In chronically-infected hosts, long-term exposure to the potent immunogens released by the miracidia within the eggs elicits a state of delayed hypersensitivity and each egg becomes the focus for the production of a granuloma.

The antigens involved in this response have been extensively studied. They appear to originate in secretory glands of the miracidia and to be released through pores in the egg shell. Homogenization of mature eggs can be used to prepare a particle-free extract containing the 'soluble egg antigens' (SEA) that initiate granuloma formation. Fractionation of SEA, using precipitation by immune mouse serum, revealed the presence of three major serological antigens, MSA1, 2 and 3. MSA1, which is a glycoprotein with a MW of 100–130 kD appears to be the most important elicitor of granulomata. As little as 1 μg will sensitize mice for granuloma formation when eggs are subsequently injected intravenously; when complexed with antibody the antigen is even more active.

The granuloma is a concentric arrangement of cells around the trapped egg (Plate 6.3). A variety of cell types are present, including macrophages, lymphocytes,

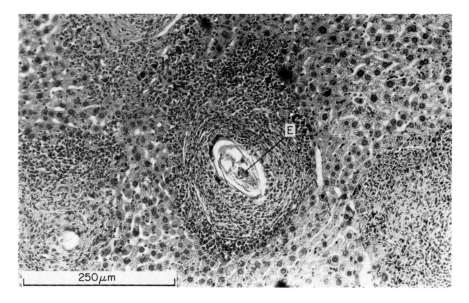

250 μm

Plate 6.3 Granuloma around the egg (E) of *Schistosoma mansoni* in the liver of a chronically infected mouse.

eosinophils, epitheloid cells and fibroblasts. Formation of the granuloma is a T cell-mediated phenomenon and can be considered as a form of DTH. Components of SEA are particularly potent in eliciting this T-cell response and some appear to be quite selective, provoking little or no antibody response. T-cell stimulation results in release of a variety of lymphokines, which initiate and regulate the granulomatous response. Among the potent material released are eosinophil chemotactic and stimulating factors, the latter enhancing bone marrow formation and release of this cell type. Eosinophils are particularly important in the reaction, since they can exert a cytotoxic function and destroy eggs.

Although granuloma formation has a primary role in initiating pathological changes, by blockage of blood vessels which leads to portal hypertension, there is also evidence that the granulomata serve a useful purpose. In suppressed or T-cell deprived mice granuloma formation is much reduced, yet mortality is increased. Around trapped eggs in the liver of such mice there are areas of necrosis and hepatocyte damage, suggestive of the release from the eggs of a hepatotoxin. If granuloma formation is protective in localizing and possibly inactivating this toxin then clearly it represents something of an over-reaction in that it leads to pathology. However, there is quite clear evidence that the degree of this over-reaction is modulated as infection progresses.

6.4.1   Modulation of Granuloma Formation

As chronic infections of mice progress beyond about 6 weeks the size of the granulomata which form around newly-trapped eggs decreases considerably (Fig. 6.9). This decrease can be shown to be correlated in time with a reduction of *in vitro* lymphocyte responsiveness to egg antigen, measured by transformation or by release of lymphokines, but with an increase in specific antibody titre. There is some evidence that the rise in antibody may contribute to the modulation in size of granulomata, but better evidence for the involvement of T-suppressor cells. Transfer of lymphocytes from 20- to 30-week infected mice (which show modulation) into 6-week infected mice (which do not) is followed by a significant reduction in the size of new granulomata. Detailed studies have implicated Lyt 2^+ cells in this suppression; removal of this population in mice with long-standing infections results in the development of larger granulomata.

Modulation of granuloma size may be seen as a finely-balanced adaptive response by the parasitized host, a balance which has some survival value. Unrestrained granuloma formation, through protecting against tissue damage from toxic factors, is clearly pathogenic, and optimization of the response is necessary to achieve protection without excessive damage. An interesting and paradoxical aspect of this balance is the effect upon the parasite, in that there is some evidence that protective responses against egg-derived toxins seem to be necessary for maximum egg release from the tissues of the host.

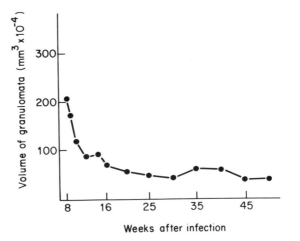

Fig. 6.9   Modulation of the granulomatous response to eggs of *Schistosoma mansoni* in the liver of infected mice. (Redrawn from Colley, 1975, *Journal of Immunology*, **115**, 150.)

7

Gastrointestinal Nematodes

Immunity within the Intestine

The vertebrate intestine can be considered one of the major ancestral sites for parasites. In evolution, access to the bodies of vertebrate hosts would have been achieved most easily through accidental ingestion. Survival in the intestine would have been favoured by the high plane of nutrition available, and the continuation of the species would have been ensured by the ready exit to the outside world. Intestinal species are, overall, still the commonest, although not the most pathogenic, of all parasites and this is seen very clearly in the nematodes. Although many species parasitize deeper tissues of the body (see Chapter 8) the majority are intestinal, and the intestine has been retained as the site of adult development even when infection occurs through skin penetration and complex tissue migrations have been incorporated into the life cycle (Fig. 7.1).

Intestinal nematodes are ubiquitous parasites of man and domestic animals (Table 7.1). The diseases they cause are rarely fatal, but instead are long-term and debilitating, their effects upon the host originating in pathological alterations of intestinal structure and function. In man such infections are common in countries where climatic and sociological conditions favour transmission, but certain species, notably the pinworm *Enterobuis vermicularis*, are equally common in the developed nations of the Western world. In domestic animals gastro-intestinal infections are invariable accompaniments of high density stocking and intensive production, and are responsible for enormous economic losses.

Many studies have shown that the intestine cannot be considered as a single habitat for parasites, but must be viewed as a series of habitats, each with its own distinctive characteristics. These characteristics change longitudinally along the length of the intestine, and also radially, from the lumen to the mucosa. Particular species have preferred locations in the intestine and are capable of active migration to such locations after infection or experimental implantation. Large worms such as *Ascaris* must necessarily live within the lumen, but smaller species such as the hookworms and trichostrongyles have an intimate association with mucosa and thus experience very different environmental conditions. Some species live within the mucosa itself during their developmental stages, emerging into the lumen when mature; a few remain wholly or partially in the mucosal tissues throughout their life in the intestine. Of these, *Trichinella spiralis* and species of *Trichuris* are thought to have intracellular locations, penetrating within the cells of the epithelial layer (Plate 7.1).

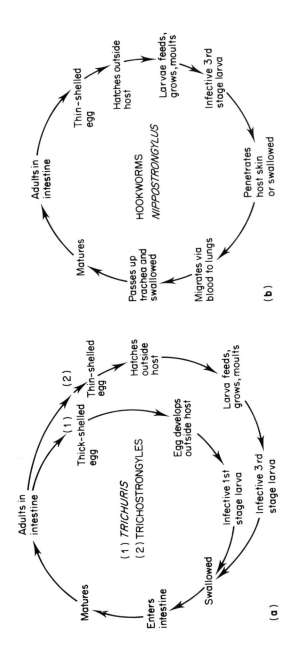

(a)

Adults in
intestine

Thick-shelled
egg
(1)

(2) Thin-shelled
egg

Hatches
outside
host

Larva feeds,
grows, moults

(1) *TRICHURIS*
(2) TRICHOSTRONGYLES

Egg develops
outside host

Infective 3rd
stage larva

Matures

Enters
intestine

Swallowed

Infective 1st
stage larva

(b)

Adults in
intestine

Thin-shelled
egg

Hatches outside
host

Larvae feeds,
grows, moults

HOOKWORMS
NIPPOSTRONGYLUS

Infective 3rd
stage larva

Matures

Passes up
trachea and
swallowed

Migrates via
blood to lungs

Penetrates
host skin
or swallowed

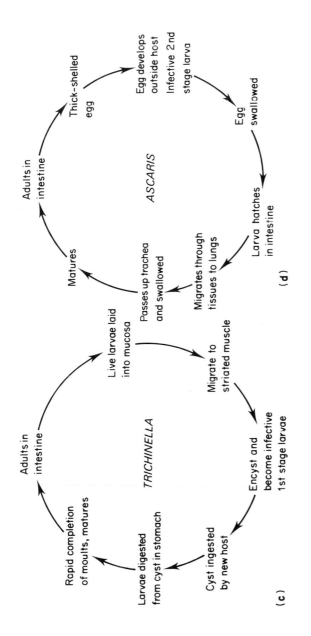

Fig. 7.1 Representative life cycles of intestinal nematodes.

Table 7.1 The major (most prevalent and/or most pathogenic) gastrointestinal nematode parasites of man and domestic animals.

Man	Cattle/sheep/pigs
Ascaris	Ascaris
Enterobius	Cooperia
Hookworms	Haemonchus
Ancylostoma	Nematodirus
Necator	Oesophagostomum
Strongyloides	Ostertagia
Trichinella	Strongyloides
Trichuris	Trichostrongylus
	Trichuris

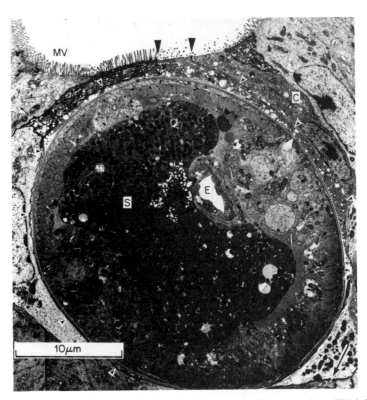

Plate 7.1 *Trichinella spiralis* within the mucosal epithelium of the mouse host. TEM showing a transverse section through the anterior end of a 24 hour-old worm, lying within an epithelial cell. C = cuticle of worm, E = oesophageal lumen, MV = microvilli on luminal surface of epithelial cell, S = stichocyte with membrane-bound α and β granules. Small arrows indicate the limits of the parasitized cell, the long arrow (bottom right) indicates the epithelial basal lamella. (Photograph from Wright, 1979, *Journal of Parasitology*, **65**, 441, by permission of the author and publishers.)

7.1 Immune Responses in the Intestine

Concepts of the operation, and even the existence, of immunity against intestinal worms were for a long time hindered by the general lack of knowledge about immune responses in the gut. Indeed it was originally proposed that worms living in the gut lumen were effectively outside the body and could neither initiate nor be affected by immune responses unless they damaged the mucosa and thereby breached what was considered to be an effective barrier. It is now known of course that this view is quite incorrect and that intestinal worms are as much subject to protective immune responses as those living elsewhere in the body. However, there are some important differences in the nature of these responses and it is necessary to outline briefly some of the characteristics of intestinal immunity before considering particular infections.

7.1.1 Antigen Uptake

The gut is a major route of entry for a variety of antigenic materials, including infectious organisms, environmental contaminants and of course food. Macromolecular uptake across the intact mucosal epithelium is a well established phenomenon. Uptake is increased when the permeability of the junctions between epithelial cells is increased (during inflammation) or when there is damage to the epithelial layer. Antigen uptake is also achieved by the activity of specialized cells in the epithelium overlying Peyer's patches. It is necessary therefore for there to be effective mechanisms to prevent wholesale swamping of the immune system and this is achieved in a variety of ways. Potential immunogens can be complexed and trapped by antibodies present at the mucosal surface. If they pass this barrier and enter the bloodstream they will be filtered out (particularly if complexed) by the liver. Intestinal presentation of antigen can be an effective means of generating non-responsiveness to antigens and this can also be seen as a means of preventing excessive immune responsiveness to ingested material.

7.1.2 Intestinal Immunoglobulins

The major isotype found at the surface of the mucosa is dimeric IgA, which can be secreted across epithelia. Large amounts also enter the intestine with bile, after secretion across bile duct epithelia. IgA remains intact and functional in the intestinal lumen by virtue of the secretory piece, which protects intra-molecular bonds from enzymatic breakdown. IgM antibodies are also transported across mucosal epithelia and similarly remain functional within the gut. IgG isotypes are produced locally, from plasma cells in the lamina propria, and may also enter the intestinal tissues from the blood. Unless the mucosa is inflamed, when both vascular and epithelial permeability increase, relatively little IgG passes into the lumen. Inflammation-induced passage of IgG into the mucosa and lumen has been termed pathotopic potentiation and may be considered as an important device to enhance resistance against intestinal pathogens. Unlike IgA and IgM, IgG molecules are rapidly degraded by proteolysis, but Fab fragments may remain intact and functional for some time. IgE is found within the intestinal mucosa but there is debate as to its origin. In some cases (e.g. the rat) there is convincing evidence that IgE is produced by plasma cells in the draining mesenteric node and transported into the lamina propria by mast cells.

Levels of complement within the mucosa are similar to those in other tissues. Some complement does enter the lumen, but it is not clear what function it can play in that site.

7.1.3   Lymphocytes

The lamina propria contains a large population of both B and T lymphocytes, the former contributing the immunoglobulins present in the mucosa and in the lumen. A specialized population of T cells, the intra-epithelial lymphocytes (IEL) is also located, as the name implies, within the epithelial layer. Their precise functions are unknown and the presence of prominent cytoplasmic granules implies a role distinct from that of the T cells within the lamina propria: a cytotoxic function is one possibility. Lamina propria T cells are known to participate in cytotoxicity and hypersensitivity reactions and their release of mediators may have an important influence upon mucosal structure and function. The Peyer's patches, which occur along the length of the intestine, are discrete units of organized lymphoid tissue, separated from the lumen by a single layer of specialized epithelial cells. One function appears to be that of sampling the luminal environment and the patches play an important initiatory role in response to antigens presented by the intestinal route.

As with systemic lymphocytes, there is a well-defined circulation of cells to and from the intestinal mucosa. Dividing cells from Peyer's patches and the draining mesenteric nodes pass into the thoracic duct lymph and selectively home, in an antigen-independent manner, back to the intestinal and other mucosal surfaces. Many of the B-cell blasts present in thoracic duct lymph are destined to become IgA-secreting plasma cells in the lamina propria; T-cell blasts enter the lamina propria and probably also contribute to the IEL population.

7.1.4   Myeloid cells

A wide variety of non-lymphoid effector cells occur within the normal intestine and their number increases during parasitic infection. These cells include natural killer cells, macrophages, neutrophils, eosinophils and basophils as well as a subset of mast cells, the mucosal mast cells. The latter, though similar to connective tissue mast cells in amine content and affinity for reaginic antibody, show several distinct properties and probably have a quite distinct origin. The infiltration of the intestine by mast cells, basophils and eosinophils shows a marked T-cell dependency. Amine release from mast cells and from basophils plays a major role in the generation of intestinal inflammation. It exerts a variety of effects upon intestinal structure and function and also influences the behaviour of the cell populations of the lamina propria. There is good evidence that hypersensitivity reactions within the mucosa influence the quantity and nature of mucus released from goblet cells and thus affect this important component of non-specific resistance in the intestine. The ways in which immunity can act against intestinal worms are shown in Fig. 7.2.

7.2   Protective Immunity against Intestinal Nematodes

Nematode parasites as a class present some particular problems for the host's protective immune response and these problems are accentuated, in the case of many intestinal species, by their remoteness from many of the immediate effectors of resistance. A major element in the pre-adaptation of nematodes to parasitism was undoubtedly their possession of a tough external cuticle. Although this is no longer considered as metabolically and immunologically inert as formerly, it nevertheless forms a substantial protective layer over the surface, being penetrated only by the mouth, anus or cloaca, female opening, excretory pore and small sensory structures (Fig. 7.3). The cuticle is both antigenic and immunogenic, but it is doubtful whether responses directed against its surface can play a major role in immunity against intestinal species. It is more likely that protective responses are initiated by antigens released through the various orifices.

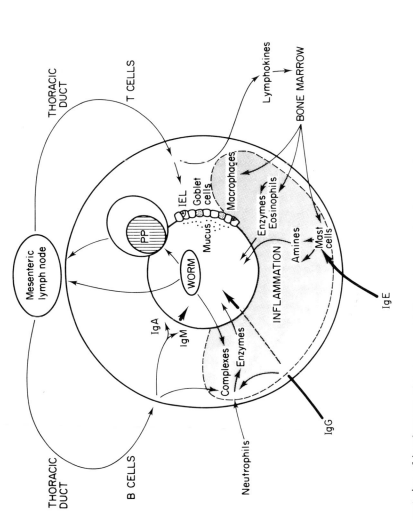

Fig. 7.2 Representation of involvement of immune and inflammatory reactions in protective responses against intestinal worms. IEL = intra epithelial lymphocytes, MLN = mesenteric lymph node, PP = Peyer's patch. (Adapted from Befus & Bienenstock, 1982, *Progress in Allergy*, **31**, 76.)

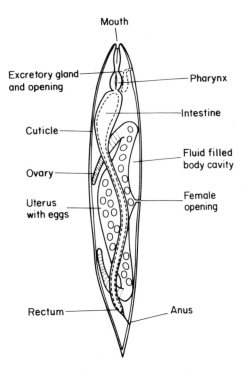

Fig. 7.3 Diagrammatic drawing of a nematode (♀) to show major structures and organ systems.

Virtually nothing is known about immunity to intestinal nematodes in man, indeed for species such as *Ascaris lumbricoides* and *Trichuris trichiura* there is evidence suggesting that immunity is non-existent. Much more is understood of immunity against these parasites in sheep and cattle, but the bulk of our detailed knowledge has come from studies made with model systems in rodents (Table 7.2). Some of these use species of nematodes that can infect man or domestic stock (*Trichinella spiralis, Trichostrongylus colubriformis*), some use related species (*Strongyloides ratti,*

Table 7.2 Species used in laboratory studies of immune responses to intestinal nematodes.

Species	Host	Cycle	
		Infection	Development
Nematospiroides dubius	Mouse	Oral – L_3	In gut
(= *Heligmosomoides polygyrus*)			Mucosa → Lumen
Nippostrongylus brasiliensis	Rat, Mouse	Skin – L_3	Migrates to gut
Strongyloides ratti	Rat, Mouse	Skin – L_3	Migrates to gut
Trichinella spiralis	Mouse, Rat, Guinea-pig	Oral – L_1	In gut
Trichostrongylus colubriformis	Guinea-pig	Oral – L_3	In gut
Trichuris muris	Mouse	Oral – L_1 in egg	In gut

Trichuris muris) and others use rodent-specific nematodes that approximate to clinically or economically-important species (*Nematospiroides dubius, Nippostrongylus brasiliensis*). Each system has distinctive features but the majority elicit a common pattern of protective responses in the intestine. With the exception of *N. dubius*, all stimulate responses that lead to expulsion of worms from the intestine during the course of a primary infection (spontaneous cure). The immunological basis and thymus dependency of spontaneous cure has been demonstrated many times and is confirmed by:

(*a*) absence of cure in T-deficient or T-deprived hosts,

(*b*) suppression of cure by treatment with immunosuppressive agents and by irradiation,

(*c*) the ability of hosts given a primary infection to express cure more rapidly on re-infection,

(*d*) transfer of the capacity to express an accelerated cure with serum or lymphocytes from immune hosts.

It has been shown in many systems that immune responses as such are but one component of the mechanism which brings about spontaneous cure and it is clear that inflammatory events also play a significant role. The importance of inflammation was emphasized as long ago as 1939, by Taliaferro and Sarles in a now classic paper describing infections with *Nippostrongylus* in rats. Their view was reinforced by observations made on 'self-cure' in sheep infected with *Haemonchus contortus*. The original experiments conducted by Stoll showed that sheep carrying an established infection of *H. contortus* expelled this infection after a superimposed infection with larval stages (Fig. 7.4) and thereafter remained refractory to further challenge for some time. Subsequent studies showed that self-cure was associated with pronounced inflammatory changes in the intestine and raised levels of histamine in the blood.

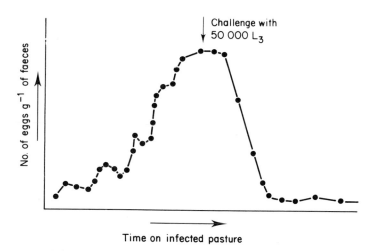

Fig. 7.4 Diagrammatic representation of 'self-cure' in sheep infected with *Haemonchus contortus*. Sheep kept on pasture contaminated with infective L₃ of *H. contortus* were allowed to build up a population of adult worms before being challenged with a heavy infection of L₃. The egg count dropped dramatically and worms were lost from the intestine.

7.2.1 Immunity against *Nippostrongylus* in the Rat

These observations directed attention towards the possible involvement of immediate hypersensitivity reactions in resistance to intestinal nematodes, and this idea has been intensively investigated using the rat–*Nippostrongylus* model (see Fig. 7.1b for life cycle). Certainly the components necessary for such reactions (i.e. reaginic antibody and mucosal mast cells) do occur in this and many other intestinal nematode infections, and indeed both can be stimulated more effectively by infection than by any other method. *Nippostrongylus* not only stimulates high levels of anti-worm IgE in the rat, it also potentiates in a non-specific way the production of IgE against many other antigens (Fig. 7.5).

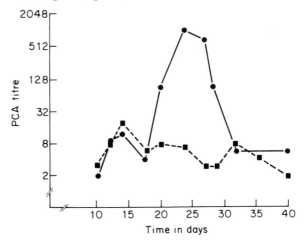

Fig. 7.5 Potentiation of anti-egg albumin IgE response in rats infected with *Nippostrongylus brasiliensis* 10 days after sensitization with egg albumin and pertussis adjuvant. Mean PCA titre in control sensitized rats (■ — — — — ■) and in infected sensitized rats (● ——————— ●) from days 10 to 40 after sensitization. (Data from Orr *et al.*, 1971, *Immunology*, **20**, 185.)

Work with *Nippostrongylus* led to three hypotheses to explain the relationship of immediate hypersensitivity to worm expulsion:

(a) amines released from mast cells damaged worms directly,

(b) intestinal inflammation resulting from amine release produced an environment unsuitable for worm survival,

(c) vascular and epithelial permeability, induced by amine release, allowed passage of anti-worm antibodies into the gut lumen (the 'leak-lesion' hypothesis, an example of pathotopic potentiation).

Evidence for and against each of these hypotheses has been presented in the literature, but there is still no consensus view. Certainly worms are damaged during the course of a primary infection, i.e. egg laying declines, cytopathological changes and lipid accumulation occur in worm tissues and there are alterations in metabolic activity and acetylcholinesterase isoenzyme patterns. During the early phase this damage is reversible, and worms survive and resume egg laying after transplantation into new hosts. Eventually the damage becomes largely irreversible and worms fail to recover after transplantation. However, loss of worms from the intestine occurs while worms are still alive and active. Evidence that amines contribute directly to this damage is tenuous and difficult to obtain experimentally using conditions that correspond to those which might occur *in vivo*. Some evidence points to a role for antibody in the induction of damage, as the characteristic features of damage occurred in worms from irradiated rats given immune serum, i.e. rats incapable of themselves mounting an active response. However, almost identical changes can be induced in worms by *in vitro* maintenance at sub-optimal conditions.

Attempts have been made to examine the importance of amine-induced inflammatory changes in spontaneous cure by inducing intestinal anaphylaxis in infected rats after sensitization to a non-parasite antigen. These attempts have been unsuccessful implying that inflammation as such (at least this particular form of inflammation) has no effect upon worm survival. An important observation made during these experiments was that worm loss did occur, if intestinal anaphylaxis was induced in rats that were then given immune serum by passive transfer (Table 7.3).

Table 7.3   Expulsion of *Nippostrongylus brasiliensis* from the intestine of rats by antiserum and induced intestinal anaphylaxis. Rats were sensitized to ovalbumin and 10 days later given 700 adult worms by laparotomy. Immune or normal serum was injected i/p after 2 days and 18 hours later the rats were injected i/v with ovalbumin to induce anaphylaxis. (Data from Barth *et al.*, 1966, *Immunology*, **10**, 459.)

Group of rats	Mean no. of worms recovered 36 h after anaphylaxis
Normal serum, no anaphylaxis	247 ± 29.4
No serum, anaphylaxis	214 ± 25.6
Immune serum, no anaphylaxis	241 ± 30.3
Immune serum, anaphylaxis	140 ± 15.3

From this observation there developed the 'leak-lesion' hypothesis (hypothesis (*c*) above), which was reinforced by later work showing a pronounced increase in mucosal permeability at the time of spontaneous cure. The authors of this hypothesis did not say that anaphylaxis was the means by which the leak lesion developed during a primary infection. Indeed they pointed out that worm-induced mucosal changes occur early in infection and 'that it is not essential to postulate an immune system-induced leak in the self (= spontaneous) cure of a primary infection' and, 'it is possible that the hypersensitive reaction functions as a rapid leak-producing system in the hyper-immune animal'. Their conclusion was that anti-worm antibody was the decisive factor in spontaneous cure, but some mechanism was required to bring antibody and worm into close contact. This mechanism could be induced directly by the worm or through release of mast cell degranulating factors.

Despite these cautious statements about the role of anaphylaxis in worm loss from a primary infection a great deal of controversy has centred around the involvement of IgE-mast cell-mediated hypersensitivity in spontaneous cure of *Nippostrongylus*. It is clear that, under certain conditions, a very suggestive correlation can be made between the rise in number of mucosal mast cells, the increase in mucosal permeability and the loss of worms, but this is not invariable. In lactating rats, for example, mucosal mastocytosis and increased permeability may occur without worm loss. In certain strains of rats, worm loss precedes the rise in mucosal mast cells. Studies on the isotype of immunoglobulin involved in passive transfer of immunity have implicated IgG, as the major Ig; sera enriched in IgE (or IgA) were ineffective. Thus, if the reagin-mast cell interaction is involved, the most that can be said is that it may contribute to spontaneous cure but it is not an essential requirement. This view is borne out by studies in mice which have shown that spontaneous cure occurs in animals rendered incapable of reagin production. In addition, though the evidence is not clear-cut, it appears that mice genetically deficient in mast cells can also expel *Nippostrongylus* in a normal time scale. One major problem in relating mast cell changes to anti-worm immunity is that much of the work carried out has used histological techniques to establish the numbers of cells present at any given time. This static picture gives no information about the dynamic changes in mast cell numbers that must accompany infection, or of the changes in content of the potent mediators that these cells contain. Indeed recent evidence shows that levels of mast cell protease correlate well with worm expulsion even when the histological picture does not.

Although passive transfer of antibody may transfer immunity against *Nippostrongylus* very effectively (Fig. 7.6) there is strong evidence that antibody by

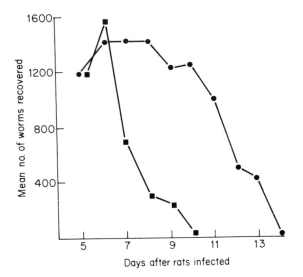

Fig. 7.6 Transfer of immunity against *Nippostrongylus brasiliensis* in rats with immune serum. ●————● untreated controls, ■————■ rats given immune serum day 4. All rats infected with 200 larvae day 0. (Redrawn from Miller, 1980, *Immunology,* **40,** 325.)

itself is not sufficient to cause worm expulsion. Other components of the immune and inflammatory response are therefore necessary. For example, irradiated rats fail to expel worms even when given antiserum of proven effectiveness (Table 7.4).

Table 7.4 Inability of antibody acting alone to bring about expulsion of *Nippostrongylus brasiliensis* from infected rats. (Data from Jones & Oglivie, 1971, *Immunology,* **20,** 549.)

Group	Irradiation	Immune Serum	Mean no. of worms recovered after 6 days
1	750 rad	6.0 ml	145 ± 49
2	None	6.0 ml	73 ± 83
3	750 rad	None	130 ± 75
4	None	None	163 ± 42

Restoration of the ability to expel worms can be conferred on sub-lethally irradiated rats by the adoptive transfer of lymphocytes if the worms concerned have already been affected by the immune response of normal rats. This was demonstrated by establishing infections by transplantation of adult worms taken from donors at a time when they would already have been damaged by the developing immunity (Table 7.5). The role played by lymphocytes in this situation is not understood, but some experiments suggest a very rapid and direct effect. Thus in rats irradiated at 750 rads and given damaged worms, the transfer of 7×10^7 T cells brought about worm loss within 5 days; other experiments suggest that both lymphocytes and myeloid cells are required for restoration of immunity in irradiated rats. Transfer of T cells (but not B cells) is also effective in intact recipients and one consequence of transfer is an accelerated appearance of mast cells in the mucosa. Whether spontaneous cure is therefore a two-step (antibody + lymphocyte) or three-step procedure (antibody + lymphocyte + myeloid cell) remains uncertain.

Table 7.5 Expulsion of 'damaged' *Nippostrongylus brasiliensis* from irradiated rats after transfer of immune lymphocytes. Rats were irradiated with 400 rads one day before receiving 700 'damaged' worms taken from donors infected 11–13 days previously. Worms were implanted by laparotomy. Immune mesenteric lymph node cells were transferred on the same day as worms were implanted. (Data from Dineen *et al.*, 1973, *International Archives of Allergy*, **45**, 504.)

	Worm recoveries 5 days after implantation	
	Geometric mean	No. of eggs/ ♀ worm
Control rats		
No cells	367	18.9
Immune cells	2	5.3
Irradiated rats		
No cells	540	15.2
Normal cells	471	14.7
Immune cells	83	7.7

7.2.2 Immunity in other Experimental Models

It is instructive to compare data gained from the *Nippostrongylus*–rat model with those obtained in other systems. Two of these in particular, *Trichinella spiralis* in the mouse and rat, and *Trichostrongylus colubriformis* in guinea pigs, have been studied in sufficient detail to make worthwhile comparisons. The latter species is a parasite of sheep which has been adapted to the guinea pig. It has a typical trichostrongyle life cycle and all parasitic stages occur within the gut lumen, close to the mucosa. Primary infections last for two to three weeks before spontaneous cure; secondary infections are expelled quickly, at about the time when the 4th larval stage is present. Immunity is transferable with serum and with lymphocytes and is strongly thymus-dependent. During infection the intestine is infiltrated by a variety of cells, of which eosinophils, basophils and mast cells are important components. There is convincing evidence to show that degranulation and amine release from basophils and mast cells play a major role in immunity. Amine levels in the gut wall and the gut lumen rise with the onset of spontaneous cure, amines can also damage worms *in vitro* and bring about worm expulsion when administered *in vivo*. Conversely, treatment of hosts with amine antagonists, or blocking agents, significantly delays worm loss. The accumulation of basophils within the mucosa is under the control of T lymphocytes and has been compared to the accumulation of these cells at sites of cutaneous basophil hypersensitivity (Jones-Mote reactions). Askenase has proposed that in such reactions there is a complex interplay between T cells, reagins, basophils and other elements. The former attract basophils to sites of antigen stimulation and, together with the interaction of antigen and reagin at the cell surface, induce amine release. The vascular permeability that results facilitates the infiltration of more basophils and other cells, notably eosinophils, thus leading to the development of a localized inflammatory response. Although in essence there is similarity with the leak-lesion hypothesis, this more complex model accounts for the involvement of more of the cell types known to be concerned with worm expulsion.

Analysis of spontaneous cure in *Trichinella spiralis* infections (see Fig. 7.1c for life cycle) has shown several significant differences from the pattern seen in the *Nippostrongylus*–rat system. Worm loss is again associated with profound inflammatory changes in the intestine, the most obvious of which are:

(*a*) infiltration of the mucosa by mast cells (Plate 7.2),
(*b*) change in fluid-flux between lumen and mucosa from net-absorption to net-secretion,
(*c*) increased peristalsis,
(*d*) villous atrophy and crypt hyperplasia.

A number of more subtle changes also occur, including alterations of brush border enzymes in epithelial cells and changes in the intestinal homing patterns of mesenteric node lymphoblasts. The result of all these changes is to make the intestine inhospitable for the worm and it has long been suggested that spontaneous cure of *Trichinella* might be brought about by such changes in the intestinal environment.

Several observations support this interpretation:

(*a*) there is a close correlation between the onset and timing of inflammation and loss of worms. This correlation is evident under a variety of experimental conditions; suppression of inflammation prevents worm expulsion;
(*b*) worms implanted directly into the gut of a mouse, whilst it is responding to a primary infection initiated by oral infection, establish for a short period but are then lost as the worms of the inducing infection are expelled;
(*c*) as with *Nippostrongylus*, worms exhibit structural and functional changes during the course of infection, but are nevertheless expelled alive. If recovered during the process of expulsion and transplanted into new hosts they survive and recover the ability to reproduce;
(*d*) the inflammation evoked by *Trichinella* is particularly potent and will remove from the intestine other parasites present concurrently.

If it is accepted that inflammatory changes are a primary cause of *Trichinella* expulsion, it is necessary to explain how these changes are generated and expressed. It is not difficult to demonstrate the immunological basis of expulsion, and immunity (accelerated expulsion) can be transferred with both serum (unreliably) and cells. Expulsion is thymus dependent and, in the mouse at least, is mediated by T lymphocytes. Cells capable of transferring immunity appear in the draining mesenteric lymph node shortly after infection and are known to be dividing cells with the phenotype of T helper cells, i.e. are Lyt $1^+ 2^-$ (Fig. 7.7). In recipients of these cells worm expulsion is accelerated by two or three days. Prior irradiation of recipients prevents expulsion after T-cell transfer, but the ability to expel worms is restored by reconstitution with bone marrow cells. This implies that non-lymphoid, bone marrow-derived cell populations have an important effector role and that these populations respond to signals derived from T-helper cells.

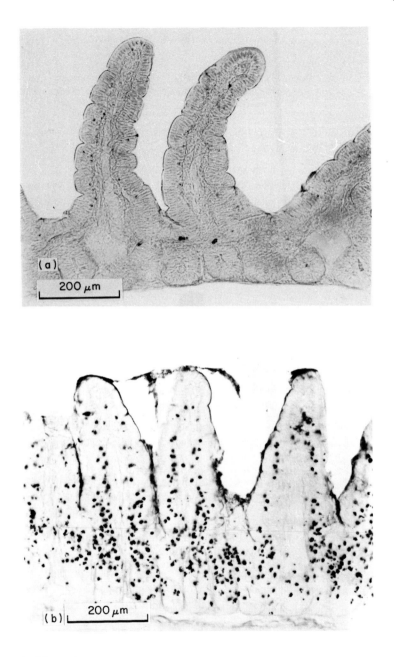

Plate 7.2 Mucosal mast cell response in the small intestine of a mouse infected with *Trichinella spiralis*. (a) Control, uninfected mouse. Very few mast cells present. (b) Mouse infected for 10 days. Extensive mastocytosis. The sections are stained with Alcian blue and safranin. The former stains the granules of the mast cells, so that cells stand out against the pale background. (Photographs by courtesy of Dr H. Alizadeh.)

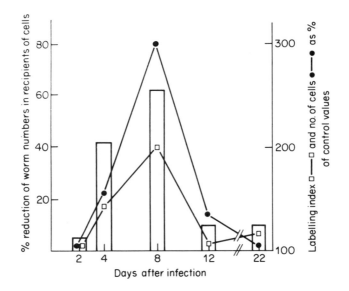

Fig. 7.7 Relations between changes in number and blast activity (labelling index) of mesenteric lymph node cells after infection of mice with *Trichinella spiralis* and the ability of the cells to transfer immunity to recipient mice. (Redrawn from Grencis & Wakelin, 1982, *Immunology*, **46**, 443.)

The increase in mucosal mast cells that accompanies infection, and the demonstration of reaginic responses, have again directed attention towards immediate hypersensitivity as a cause of spontaneous cure. There is some evidence that immunity can be transferred with sera enriched in IgE, but, as with *Nippostrongylus* it is not always possible to correlate mast cell responses with worm expulsion. However, as discussed above, the functional role of mast cells may not necessarily be related to the numbers of cells detectable by routine histological techniques. The very obvious infiltration of the mucosa by these cells is indicative of a pronounced inflammatory response, and it is hard to resist the conclusion that some facet of mast cell function must contribute to the total expulsion response under normal conditions. This contribution is, however, not essential and the other components of inflammation can bring about worm expulsion equally well in its absence. Mast cells are but one cell type found in increased numbers in the infected gut, both neutrophils and eosinophils are present and there is also an increase in goblet cells. Measurement of enzymes associated with leucocytes, and specifically with eosinophils, e.g. myeloperoxidases and phospholipases, has shown marked increases in levels in the lumen and mucosa at the time of worm expulsion. Again these observations demonstrate correlative, rather than causal, connections but support the view that overall inflammatory changes do bring about expulsion.

It is relevant to ask whether directly expressed anti-worm immunity has any part to play in resistance to *Trichinella*. In the mouse, transfer of B cell-enriched fractions of immune lymphocyte populations does not induce an accelerated worm expulsion. Nevertheless there is transfer of an immunity that is measurable in reduced growth and fecundity. It is probable that this anti-worm immunity may reflect the effects of an antibody-mediated interference with feeding. If this is the case, the affected worms would be less active metabolically and perhaps less able to maintain themselves in an environment that becomes progressively less suitable for their survival. The successful passive transfer of immunity with serum might therefore be interpreted as bringing about sub-optimal viability of worms, making them prematurely susceptible to the T cell-mediated inflammatory changes. Clearly this is an oversimplification. IgA antibodies are known to reduce worm fecundity *in vitro*, a situation in which interference with feeding seems less likely. In addition anti-worm antibodies may interact with free antigen and complement to initiate inflammatory changes and also be involved in enhancing the development of mastocytosis.

As with all systems, experience of a primary infection with *Trichinella* generates strong immunity to re-infection. In the mouse this is normally expressed as an accelerated version of the primary spontaneous cure, but under certain conditions there can be a very rapid expulsion of challenge larvae, the majority of worms being lost within 24 hours. In rats rapid expulsion is the normal response to re-infection. One explanation for this phenomenon is trapping of larvae in mucus, thus preventing access to the mucosa and allowing removal of worms by peristalsis (Table 7.6). It may be that antibody in the mucus plays a part in this trapping, perhaps through interaction with antigens present on the cuticle, but there is little evidence for this at present. Mucus trapping is not the whole explanation of rapid expulsion as some challenge larvae do reach the mucosa and the majority of these are also expelled rapidly. Of the pathological changes which accompany the loss of primary infections, only the change in epithelial cells leading to net fluid secretion into the lumen can be identified during rapid expulsion. One possiblity is that epithelial changes render the cells unsuitable for occupancy by the worms. The speed of rapid expulsion is suggestive of a hypersensitivity reaction and there are certain attractions in this hypothesis. It has been amply demonstrated that such reactions can stimulate a release of increased amounts of mucus from goblet cells, and numbers of goblet cells increase during primary infection and remain elevated for a considerable time. Unfortunately attempts to block rapid expulsion by treatment of the host with drugs known to inhibit or block immediate hypersensitivity reactions have proved unsuccessful. Mucus trapping may well be a widespread phenomenon in resistance to helminth infections, recent evidence suggests that it contributes to immunity to *Nippostrongylus* in rats and to *Haemonchus contortus* in sheep.

7.3 Antigens Involved in Immunity

Although in general little is known of the antigens that stimulate protective responses against intestinal nematodes, considerable progress has been made with *Trichinella spiralis*. Detailed studies have been made of antigens present at the cuticular surface (see Chapter 8) and of antigens released from the stichosome. At present there is no evidence to implicate the former in intestinal immunity but there is very good evidence that the latter are functional in this respect.

In *Trichinella*, as in all members of the Trichinelloidea (e.g. *Trichuris*), the oesophagus is a duct of very narrow diameter, embedded for the greater part of its length in a chain of large cylindrical cells, the stichocytes. Collectively the structure forms the stichosome. The cytoplasm of the stichocytes is rich in membrane-bound α and β granules (see Plate 7.1) which, it is believed, pass into the oesophagus through narrow ducts. The contents of the granules are released from the mouth and can be collected in soluble form from culture fluids in which worms have been maintained. The precise functions of the granules are unknown although it seems reasonable to assume that they have a role in penetration of epithelial cells and/or in extra-corporeal digestion of tissues for feeding. This view is supported by the fact that the granule contents of the infective muscle larvae are released within the first 24 hours after entry into the intestine and are then resynthesized.

Table 7.6 Mucus trapping of infective larvae of *Trichinella spiralis* after infection of immune rats. Differential recovery procedures were used to count larvae present at different levels between lumen and epithelial layer of intestine. (Data from Lee & Ogilvie, 1981, In *Trichinellosis*, ed. Kim, Ruitenberg & Teppema, Reedbooks, England.)

Time after infection	Group	Total larval recovery	Free in lumen	No. of larvae recovered as % of total		
				Superficial mucus globules	Intermediate layer of mucus	Deep mucus and epithelium
90 minutes	Control	1875	11	2	4	83
	Immune	1942	3	56	2	39
3 hours	Control	2033	21	2	5	72
	Immune	1628	27	41	2	31

Granule fractions prepared by density-gradient centrifugation of larval homogenates, and secretions released by larvae into *in vitro* maintenance media are highly immunogenic. Injection of as little as 50 μg of granule material into mice elicits an immunity that is expressed in an accelerated rejection of a challenge infection. In amounts of 10 μg or less, immunity is seen primarily as a reduction in worm size and fecundity (Fig. 7.8). Analysis of granule extracts by electrophoretic and iso-electric focussing techniques has revealed a complex mixture of proteins and glycoproteins, but there is evidence that particular components are immunogenic *in vivo*.

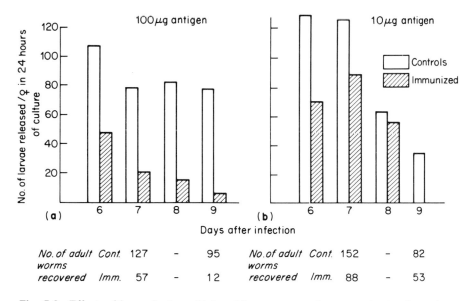

Fig. 7.8 Effects of immunization with larval homogenate antigen upon *in vitro* fecundity (graphs) and survival of adult *Trichinella spiralis* in mice. Antigen given in CFA as 3 injections at weekly intervals, mice infected with 200 larvae 1–2 weeks after the last injection. (Data from Despommier *et al.*, 1977, *Parasitology*, **74**, 109.)

The knowledge now available of *Trichinella* antigens makes it possible to devise a scheme to explain the manifestations of immunity seen during the primary infection. Release of stichosomal antigen into the mucosa would lead to the proliferation of lymphocytes in the mesenteric node. Blast cells would then migrate back to the small intestine via the thoracic duct. B cell blasts would differentiate into plasma cells and secrete antibody of various isotypes. T-cell blasts would proliferate and release a variety of factors that initiate cell infiltration, mucosal mastocytosis and functional changes in mucosal structure. Antibody would combine with secreted antigen, forming immune complexes, thus inactivating the granule contents and possibly thereby restricting feeding. As a result worms would develop cytopathological changes and female worms would lose their ability to produce larvae. Immune complexes might also initiate inflammatory reactions (Type III hypersensitivity). Inflammation would be increased by the activities of the cells attracted by T cell and other factors. Eventually the immediate environment of the worms would become so inhospitable that the worms would leave the mucosa and be removed by rapid peristalsis of the fluid-filled gut contents.

7.4   Chronic Infections

The model systems described above are characterized by the development of strong immune responses which are effective against the worms of a primary infection and give good protection against re-infections. Clearly, if this was typical of all intestinal nematode infections they would not present the problems that they do. In man and domestic stock gastro-intestinal nematodes are characteristically associated with chronic and often intense infections and for the majority there is little obvious evidence of an effective immunity. Circumstantial evidence suggests that immunity may occur with some species, for example in human hookworms, where infection levels plateau in the older members of the population. However there is no evidence for strong spontaneous cure responses. Thus although some model systems provide valuable information about the ways in which intestinal responses can control intestinal nematodes, other experimental systems are necessary to discover why such responses are inoperative or ineffective in many cases.

Failure to generate effective responses may have many explanations and unless detailed epidemiological data are available, it cannot automatically be assumed that chronic infections reflect total inability to develop resistance. For example, one important consideration is the level and frequency of infection. In the laboratory it is customary to use relatively large, single pulse infections in order to establish workable models; in the field such infections would normally be the exception, instead hosts are likely to be exposed to continuous. or interrupted, low level 'trickle' infections. It has been shown with *Nippostrongylus* that trickle infections can produce large and persistent infections, i.e. the normal spontaneous cure response does not occur (Fig. 7.9). Rats given 5 larvae per day for 12 weeks accumulated approximately 100 worms, 30% of the total infection. This is lower than the average 50% establishment recorded after single large pulse infections and a proportion of trickle worms were stunted in growth. These facts indicate some development of immunity and this is confirmed by the ability of trickle-infected rats to expel subsequent large challenge infections. When rats were infected with 50 larvae per day there was a partial expulsive response, but stunted worms continued to establish and a substantial population accumulated. Worms can also be established in immune rats

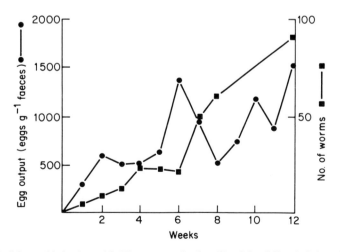

Fig. 7.9   Build-up of infection with *Nippostrongylus brasiliensis* by daily administration of 5 infective larvae to rats. (Redrawn from Jenkins & Phillipson, 1970, *Parasitology*, **62**, 457.)

by means of trickle infection. As before, these worms are stunted and less fecund but do survive. A great deal of evidence points to the fact that worms maturing from trickle infections adapt in some way to the immune responses they elicit, becoming both less immunogenic and less susceptible to immune responses when these are provoked by conventional pulse infections.

Work with *Nippostrongylus* has also shown that the normal pattern of spontaneous cure fails to develop in rats infected when very young, i.e. less than 6 weeks old, and worm burdens may persist into adult life. This situation has significant parallels with gastro-intestinal worm infections in sheep, and of course may be relevant to man, as young children are most at risk from infection. However, the extent to which such experimental findings can be extrapolated has yet to be determined. What is true of *Nippostrongylus* in the rat is certainly not true of all model systems. For example it has been shown with *Trichuris muris* in mice that the spontaneous cure response cannot be circumscribed by either trickle or neonatal infections.

7.4.1 Chronic Infections in Experimental Models

In addition to the factors discussed above, it is known that genetic and nutritional influences affect the host's capacity to respond protectively to infection. It is also well established that immunity to intestinal worms can be depressed when the host is concurrently infected with other infectious agents, including other species of nematodes. However, even when all these considerations can be ruled out, as is possible in the laboratory, there still remain species which seem not to evoke effective responses in the host. One such parasite, which has proved a fruitful model for the study of chronic infections is *Nematospiroides dubius* (known also as *Heligmosomoides polygyrus*). This worm has a typical trichostrongyle life cycle, but the larvae spend approximately 8 days within the gut wall before emerging and maturing as adults in the gut lumen. When mice are given a primary infection with this species, the adult worms may persist for as long as 8 months, and their eventual loss seems to owe more to senility than to immune expulsion. In the majority of mouse strains, challenge infections develop as successfully as the preceding primary and do not seem to be greatly affected by immunity.

Despite this evidence for long term survival it is possible to show that there are substantial immune responses elicited by infection and, under appropriate conditions, these can be seen to be protective. One way of achieving immunity is to repeatedly infect mice, removing the adult burdens at intervals to prevent a lethal accumulation of worms in the intestine. Under these conditions it can be seen that progressively fewer challenge larvae mature as adults and eventually complete resistance is achieved. Protective responses are also stimulated by infection with larvae that have been irradiated at 25 krad and are therefore incapable of completing the mucosal phase of development. When mice immunized in this way are challenged with normal larvae, the larvae become trapped in the mucosa and are destroyed (Fig. 7.10). These experiments point to the mucosal larvae as the immunogenic phase and as the target for immune effector mechanisms. The development of inflammatory granulomata around trapped larvae suggests that some form of antibody-dependent-cell-mediated cytotoxicity (ADCC) may be involved.

If mice can generate such effective immunity under chemotherapy or after infection with irradiated larvae the question arises as to why immunity is not generated or expressed when normal infections are given. A significant pointer to one reason is given by experiments in which mice are concurrently infected with both irradiated and normal larvae. The latter develop into adult worms and the mice remain susceptible to challenge.

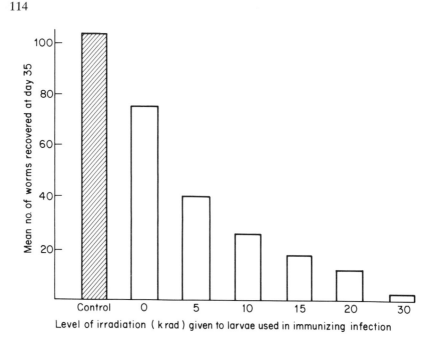

Fig. 7.10 Stimulation of immunity against *Nematospiroides dubius* in mice. Mice were given 200 normal or irradiated larvae, treated with anthelmintic on days 34 and 35 and challenged after 42 days with 100 normal larvae. (Redrawn from Hagan *et al.*, 1981, *Parasite Immunology*, **3**, 149.)

It can only be concluded that normal larvae and/or adult worms in some way suppress the initiation or expression of the immunity that the irradiated larvae would otherwise produce. Direct evidence that it is the adults which exert this effect comes from experiments in which adult worms were implanted directly into the intestine before infection with irradiated larvae. Under these conditions the irradiated larvae stimulated no immunity (Fig. 7.11). Similarly, when primary infections are terminated as soon as worms emerge into the lumen, the mice are strongly resistant to challenge whereas mice in which adult worms have been allowed to persist remain susceptible.

The mechanisms of this suppression by adult worms are uncertain. It is known that mice infected with *N. dubius* show depressed responsiveness to a variety of unrelated antigens, including SRBC, influenza virus and other intestinal nematodes. Mice concurrently harbouring *N. dubius* and *T. spiralis* fail to develop or express immunity against the latter. *N. dubius* infection also interferes with the adoptive transfer of immunity against *T. spiralis* but this effect is reversed when *N. dubius* is removed by chemotherapy. This shows that lymphocytes with *T. spiralis* specificity survive intact, but are in some way prevented from generating an effective anti-*T. spiralis* response when *N. dubius* is present. Recent work has shown that the depression of SRBC responses in *N. dubius* infected mice is associated with impairment of macrophage function in antigen presentation and with the appearance of suppressor T cells. Suppression can also be induced effectively by intravenous injection of adult worm homogenate.

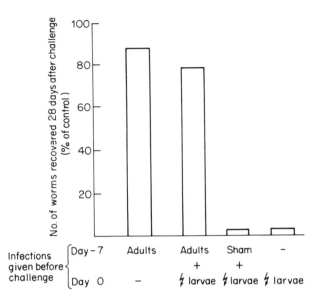

Infections given before challenge	Day – 7	Adults	Adults	Sham	–
			+	+	
	Day 0	–	⚡ larvae	⚡ larvae	⚡ larvae

Fig. 7.11 Suppression of immunity against *Nematospiroides dubius* in mice by adult worms. Mice were given 100 adults by laparotomy and/or 200 irradiated larvae. Worms were removed by anthelmintic on days 42 and 44 and the mice challenged with 200 normal larvae on day 49. (Redrawn from Behnke *et al.*, 1983, *Parasite Immunology*, **5**, 397.)

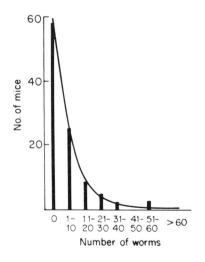

Fig. 7.12 Overdispersion of infection. The numbers of mature pinworms (*Aspiculuris tetraptera*) recovered from a wild population of female house mice. (Data from Behnke, 1975, *Journal of Helminthology*, **49**, 85.)

7.4.2   Biological Significance of Chronic Infections

In biological terms chronic infections, however achieved, undoubtedly favour parasite survival, since they allow prolonged reproductive activity. It is not necessary that all members of the population carry chronic infections, merely that enough do so to maintain an adequate rate of transmission to susceptible individuals. One of the striking aspects of parasite distribution in natural populations, including man, is that there is overdispersion (Fig. 7.12), i.e. the majority of hosts have few parasites, and the majority of parasites occur in few hosts. It may well be that these heavily and chronically-infected individuals maintain transmission of the parasite concerned and thus ensure its survival. Genetically-determined differences between individuals in susceptibility, or in ability to develop resistance, certainly do contribute to overdispersion, but many other factors are also important. Immunity to gastro-intestinal nematodes seems to operate relatively inefficiently in young animals and it is also very effectively depressed by the physiological changes which accompany pregnancy and lactation, particularly the latter. As a result, reproductively active females provide an important source of infection for their susceptible young, who may then respond ineffectively and become chronically infected. In sheep parasitized by gastro-intestinal trichostrongyles, parturition and lactation are associated with a marked elevation of faecal egg output (the Spring Rise) as immunity is depressed and larval nematodes, whose development has been inhibited, become mature. It is difficult to disentangle the effects of this proven depression of immunity from the environmentally-induced diapause-like condition that many trichostrongyles enter over winter. Nevertheless, the net effect is to contaminate pasture heavily with infective larval stages, ensuring transmission to new born lambs, and promoting survival of the parasite. The chronic intestinal infections of man may similarly reflect the operation of successful survival strategies by the worms concerned.

8

Nematodes which Invade Tissues
The Cuticle as Target for Effector Mechanisms

8.1   Protective Immune Responses
8.2   Responses against Larvae in Blood and other Tissues
8.3   Hypersensitivity and Immunopathology

Exploitation of habitats other than those provided by the intestine of the host is widespread in the Nematoda. Many species that live as adults in the intestine, e.g. *Ascaris*, hookworms, *Nippostrongylus* and *Trichinella*, undergo development in parenteral tissues. Other species are wholly confined to the tissues and have no contact with the intestine. The occupation of such niches within the body requires particular adaptations in reproductive biology, the parasite concerned no longer having direct access to the outside world. One way of solving this problem (seen in *Capillaria* and *Trichinella*) is the production of stages, eggs or cysts, which remain infective in the tissues after the death of the host or which are infective when the host is eaten. Another (seen in *Dracunculus*) is to break out of the surface of the body in order to liberate larvae. In a major group of tissue-invading nematodes, the Filarioidea, the problem is solved by the involvement of a blood-feeding arthropod intermediate host in the life cycle (Fig. 8.1). The female worms liberate live embryos – microfilaria larvae – which circulate in the blood or accumulate in the skin. The arthropod takes up microfilariae when it feeds, provides an environment in which development to infectivity can occur, and then re-introduces the parasite into the vertebrate host at a subsequent blood meal. For the major filarial infections of man the intermediate hosts are as follows:

Lymphatic filariases: *Wuchereria bancrofti, Brugia malayi* – transmitted by species of mosquito.

Onchocerciasis: *Onchocerca volvulus* – transmitted by species of *Simulium*.
However, many other arthropods, including ticks and mites can also transmit worms of this group.

In several species of filarial worms there is an intricate interrelationship between the behavioural patterns of parasite and vector, which results in an optimization of the uptake of microfilarial stages. The latter are not present in peripheral blood throughout the 24 hour cycle but appear for limited periods during the day or during the night. The periodicity of the parasite coincides with the time at which the vector feeds most actively. In *Wuchereria bancrofti*, for example, the microfilaria larvae appear in the peripheral blood for an hour or two each side of midnight, when the mosquito is feeding. For the remainder of the 24 hours the larvae remain within the deep organs of the body, particularly the lungs, actively maintaining position against the flow of blood. Movement into and out of peripheral blood is controlled by the physiological rhythms of the host and is reversed if the waking-sleeping pattern of the host is reversed.

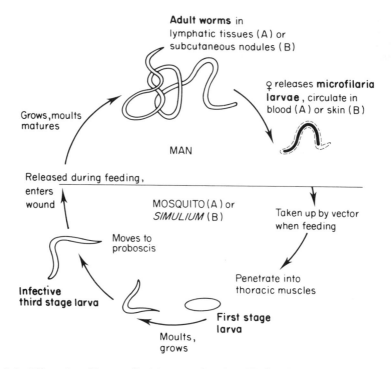

Fig. 8.1 Life cycles of human filarial nematodes. A = *Wuchereria* or *Brugia*, B = *Oncho-cerca*. The life cycles of the common laboratory models *Brugia pahangi* and *Dipetalonema viteae* are similar to A. *D. viteae* adults lie unencapsulated below the skin and their larvae are transmitted by ticks.

Filarial infections are responsible for some of the most important parasitic diseases of man and they are endemic in areas which allow the development of suitable intermediate hosts (Table 8.1). All are long-term, chronic diseases, characterized by morbidity rather than by mortality. They are associated with debilitating

Table 8.1 Filarial infections of man.

Species	Vector	Occurrence	Pathogenicity
Wuchereria bancrofti	Mosquito	Many countries in tropics/sub-tropics	Mild/severe Lymphoid/skin
Brugia malayi	Mosquito	Asia	Mild/severe Lymphoid/skin
Loa loa	Tabanid flies	Africa	Mild
Mansonella ozzardi	Midges	C. and S. America	Benign
Dipetalonema perstans	Midges	Africa, C. and S. America	Benign
D. streptocara	Midges	Africa	Benign
Onchocerca volvulus	*Simulium,* blackflies	Africa, C. and S. America	Severe Lymphoid/skin/ eyes

pathological changes, particularly in the lymphoid system and in the skin. Swelling and inflammation of the lymph nodes occur commonly with all three species listed above; inflammation and blockage of lymphatics is characteristic of *Wuchereria* and *Brugia*. Changes in the skin and dermal tissues are most pronounced in onchocerciasis and this infection also leads to severe eye lesions and the loss of sight. Both lymphatic species may induce skin and dermal changes in the condition known as elephantiasis. Pathology in onchocerciasis is due entirely to the microfilarial stage, in the lymphatic species it is primarily the adult worms that are harmful. It is known that many of the changes associated with filarial infection are immunopathological in origin and that hypersensitivity reactions are particularly important in their development. It must be remembered, however, that not all human filarial infections are severely pathogenic, a number are quite benign despite their chronicity and give rise to very few clinical symptoms.

The existence of immunopathological changes in filarial disease reflects the close and intimate contact between tissue-dwelling worms and the immunological mechanisms of the host. Parasite antigens are freely available to the host and, unlike gastro-intestinal species, the worms are readily accessible to effector agents such as antibody, complement and cytotoxic cells. It is therefore possible to think of immunity against such worms in conventional terms, the direct interactions between effectors and the worm playing a major role. It might be thought that, under these conditions, host responses would constitute an effective barrier to successful parasitism, but clearly this is not the case. Filarial nematodes are not only large and successful parasites, infecting an estimated 300 million people, but their life span is considerable, individual worms surviving for many years in the host. *Onchocerca volvulus*, for example lives for more than 15 years. This long-term survival is the more remarkable when it is apparent that infections do elicit strong immune responses, most characteristically reflected in raised levels of IgE and pronounced eosinophilia.

8.1 Protective Immune Responses

The chronicity of filarial infections implies either that protective responses are absent or weak, or that worms evade such responses by reducing their immunogenicity or by suppressing the host. A number of facts point to the existence of protective immunity but, as with other parasite infections the evidence in man is essentially circumstantial and derives from epidemiological observations that infection levels plateau or decline with age (Fig. 8.2), even though there is continuing transmission. *In vitro* studies, using human cells and sera, have also shown the existence of antibodies capable of mediating cytotoxic responses against parasite stages (see below). Experimental investigation of *in vivo* mechanisms of immunity against the filarial species that infect man is hindered by the rigid host specificity which the majority show. However, related species can be maintained in laboratory hosts and these, together with rodent species, provide valuable models for studying both those situations in which effective protective responses do develop and those in which immunity appears ineffective (Table 8.2). In the former, immunity is evident in the death of adult worms or in their loss of fecundity, in clearance of microfilariae from the blood stream and in the failure of challenge infections to become fully established. In the latter, ineffective immunity is reflected in an inability to resist challenge infections even when repeatedly infected over long periods of time (Fig. 8.3). Both types of models have thrown light on mechanisms involved in resistance.

Many studies of protective immunity have concentrated upon responses directed against microfilarial stages, as these are amenable to *in vitro* manipulation. Analyses of responses against the infective and adult stages present more difficult technical problems. The mechanisms by which hosts may protect themselves against filarial

120

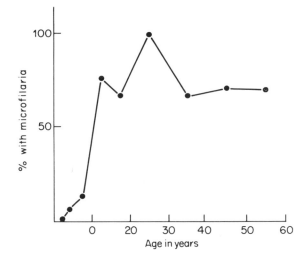

Fig. 8.2 Prevalence of *Onchocerca* in a population living in an endemic area of Africa. (Data from Duke & Moore, 1968, *Transactions of the Royal Society for Tropical Medicine and Hygiene*, **62**, 22.)

Table 8.2 Laboratory model systems used for studying immunity to filarial infections.

Species	Host
Onchocerca spp.	Cow, Horse, (Mouse)
Brugia malayi	Rhesus monkey, Cat, Jird
Brugia pahangi	Cat, Jird, Rat, (Mouse)
Dirofilaria immitis	Dog
Dipetalonema viteae	Jird, Hamster, (Mouse)
Litomosoides carinii	Cotton rat

(Mouse) signifies use of host for establishment of infection by direct transfer of adult worms, injection of microfilariae, or after immunological manipulation.

parasites present in tissues can also be studied using heterologous models such as *Trichinella*, which has a major parenteral phase in its life cycle. The relative simplicity of this model has allowed substantial progress to be made in understanding host-parasite interactions as they relate to tissue nematodes and it will be considered in some detail.

8.2 Responses against Larvae in Blood and other Tissues

It has been shown repeatedly, both in man and in experimental hosts, that filarial infections are associated with production of antibodies directed against the cuticle of the microfilariae. These antibodies can be detected and quantified by immunofluorescence or by their ability to mediate adherence of cells to the larvae. Two observations in particular have focussed attention upon the role of such antibodies in host-protective responses. Firstly, in many cases, antibodies with

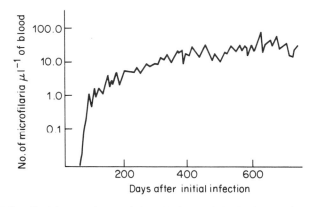

Fig. 8.3 Microfilarial counts in a cat infected with 200 infective larvae of *Brugia pahangi* on day 0 and reinfected, after 136 days, with 50 larvae at intervals of about 10 days. At *post-mortem* examination a total of 128 adults worms was recovered. (Redrawn from Denham *et al.*, 1972, *International Journal of Parasitology*, **2**, 401.)

specificity for the microfilarial cuticle do not appear until after the host becomes amicrofilaraemic i.e. when larvae are no longer detectable in the blood (Fig. 8.4). Anti-microfilarial antibodies therefore correlate much better with resistance than do those against infective larvae or adult worms. Secondly, antibody-mediated cell adherence has been shown to be cytotoxic and to result in the death of larvae. By implication the antigens which elicit these responses must be present at the surface of the cuticle, and the effector mechanisms which destroy the larvae must do so by damaging the cuticular layer in the first instance. Both of these assumptions have been amply confirmed in several studies with filarial species, but have been most completely studied using *Trichinella* as a model system.

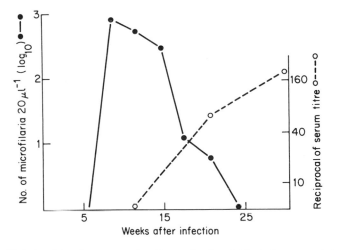

Fig. 8.4 Relationship between microfilaraemia in LAKZ hamsters infected with *Dipetalonema viteae* and appearance of antibodies with specificity for microfilarial surface antigens. Titre of serum antibody measured using indirect immunofluorescence. (Data from Weiss, 1978, *Acta Tropica*, **35**, 137.)

8.2.1   Responses against *Trichinella* larvae

The newborn larvae of *Trichinella* resemble microfilariae in three important respects:
(*a*) they are relatively undifferentiated,
(*b*) they are liberated directly by the female worm into host tissues,
(*c*) they undergo extensive migration in the tissues.
Newborn larvae have the additional advantage that they are easily obtained in large quantities by *in vitro* maintenance of adult worms and therefore make good experimental material.

Initial studies, using serum from rats exposed to complete infections with *Trichinella*, showed the presence of antibodies capable of recognizing antigens present on the cuticles of all three major life-cycle stages, namely infective larva, adult and newborn larva (Fig. 8.5). Cross absorption studies, using living worms, confirmed the stage-specificity of the antibodies, from which it was inferred that stage-specific antigens were present on the cuticular surface. Antibody-mediated cell adherence occurred with all three stages (Plate 8.1) and, in the case of newborn larvae, could rapidly inactivate and destroy the worm. Adherence and killing were primarily antibody dependent, though enhanced when complement was present, and killing required the presence of eosinophils and macrophages. Subsequent work has shown, as with schistosomula larvae of schistosomes, that the eosinophil major basic protein is a particularly effective agent in bringing about disintegration of the larval cuticle and subsequent destruction of internal organs. The cuticle of freshly released newborn larvae does not activate complement, but this property is acquired after about 24 hours of culture *in vitro* and is then retained by both the muscle larval and adult stages.

The antigens responsible for the production of anticuticular antibodies have been localized and characterized using the techniques developed for radio-labelling of proteins in cell membranes (Fig. 8.6). In these techniques, live worms are incubated with reagents that couple isotopes to lysine or tyrosine within protein-containing molecules present at the cuticular surface. The labelled worms are then homogenized to release the labelled molecules and the homogenate is electrophoresed on polyacrylamide gels to resolve the components. An autoradiograph is prepared to reveal labelled bands on the gel. Further information can be gained by interpolating an additional step before electrophoresis in order to precipitate components of the homogenate by antibodies known to be directed against cuticular targets.

The results of this work have shown that each stage in the developmental cycle of *Trichinella* possesses a restricted and characteristic set of surface antigens. Those of the newborn larvae comprise two pairs of antigens with apparent molecular weights of 64 kD and 58 kD, and 30 kD and 28 kD (Plate 8.2). The four antigens of the infective larvae, which can be prepared in greater quantity, share a common polypeptide back-bone, but differ in being monomeric or dimeric, and in the presence or absence of a carbohydrate component. There is evidence that these antigens are released from the cuticle into the medium when worms are cultured *in vitro*, i.e. there appears to be a continuous turnover of material. The origin of the antigens and the manner in which they are presented at the surface of the cuticle and then released are at present unknown.

8.2.2   Responses against Microfilariae

Using techniques similar to these outlined above, surface antigens have been identified on microfilariae of a number of filarial nematodes, including *W. bancrofti*, *B. malayi*, *B. pahangi*, *O. volvulus* and *D. viteae*. As with *Trichinella*, these antigens

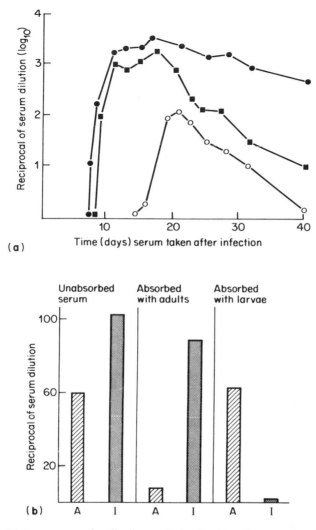

Fig. 8.5 (a) Appearance of antibodies mediating *in vitro* adherence of peritoneal exudate cells to stages of *Trichinella spiralis* after infection of rats. ● = infective larvae, ■ = adults worms, ○ = newborn larvae. Sera were taken at intervals, inactivated and used for *in vitro* culture of worms with non-adherent peritoneal exudate cells. (b) Stage specificity of antibodies mediating cell adherence. 14 day serum was absorbed with either adults or infective larvae and used for cell adherence against these stages. A = Adult, I = Infective larvae. In both (a) and (b) the end-point of the assay was the serum dilution at which 50% of the worm's surface was covered by cells. (Data from Mackenzie *et al.*, 1978, *Nature*, **276**, 826.)

are restricted in heterogeneity, but they are not as completely stage specific, showing cross reactivity between different developmental stages of the same species. In addition there is cross reactivity between similar stages of different species. Antibodies to these surface antigens mediate cell adherence to microfilariae and this adherence can result in killing of the worm. *In vitro* adherence and cytotoxicity have

124

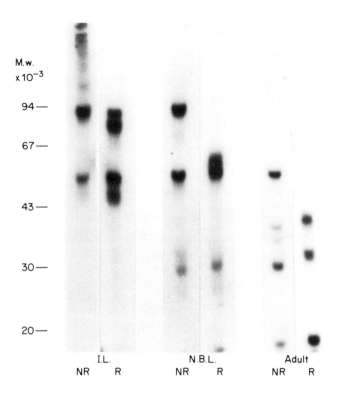

M.w.
x10⁻³

94 —

67 —

43 —

30 —

20 —

I.L.   N.B.L.   Adult
NR   R   NR   R   NR   R

Plate 8.1 Surface antigens of three stages of *Trichinella spiralis*. After surface labelling using radioactive iodide and chloramine T, worms were homogenized and the homogenates processed as described in the text (Fig. 8.6). The bands obtained by analysis using SDS–PAGE are shown for the infective larval (IL), new born larval (NBL) and adult stages under non-reducing (NR) and reducing (R) conditions. The position of molecular weight markers run in parallel is shown on the left hand side of the figure. Under reducing conditions the major bands obtained were: IL – 105, 90, 55 and 47 kD, NBL – 64, 58, 34 and 30 kD, Adult – 40, 33 and 20 kD. (Photograph from Clark *et al.*, 1982, *Biochemical Journal*, **206**, 27, by permission of the author and publishers.)

been extensively studied using antibodies known to have general surface specificity, but there have as yet been few studies using antibodies with specificity for particular surface antigens.

As with ADCC against schistosomula, a variety of Ig classes and of effector cells appear to be effective against microfilariae. IgG-mediated adherence of human leucocytes (including eosinophils) has been described using *W. bancrofti* and *O. volvulus*. IgM-mediated adherence of neutrophils and macrophages has been reported with *D. viteae* in the hamster, and IgE-mediated adherence of eosinophils and macrophages occurs with *D. viteae* in the rat. The essential role of the cellular elements in killing was elegantly demonstrated by experiments in which microfilariae of *D. viteae* were placed within micropore chambers, which were in turn implanted into immune hamsters. When chambers with a pore size of 0.3 μm were used, no cells were able to enter the chambers and the larvae survived for at least 3 weeks. When chambers with a pore size of 3 or 5 μm were used, cells entered the chambers and the

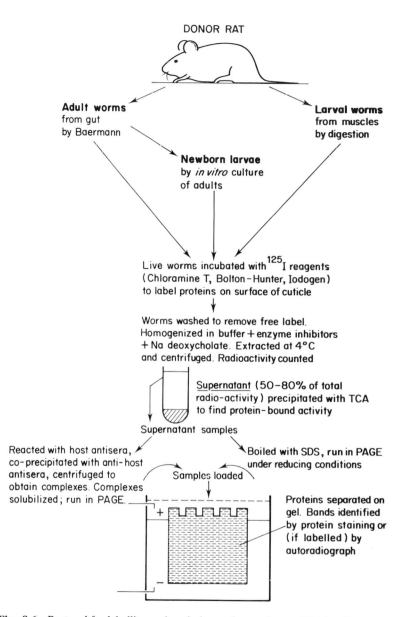

Fig. 8.6 Protocol for labelling and analysing surface antigens of *Trichinella spiralis*. (Based on Parkhouse *et al.*, 1981, *Parasite Immunology*, **3**, 339.)

larvae were dead within 24 hours. The same result was obtained when microfilariae were pre-incubated in the IgM fraction of immune serum before being placed in 3 μm pore size chambers and implanted into normal hamsters (Table 8.3). This *in vitro* evidence for interaction between IgM and leucocytes is supported by *in vivo* data gained from using a strain of mice (CBA/n) genetically incapable of making IgM

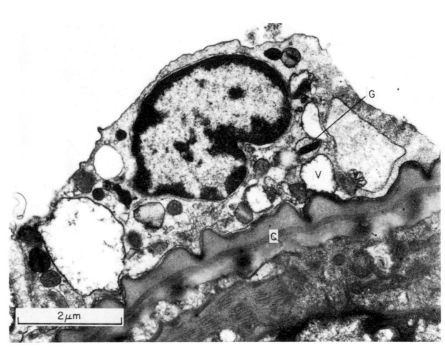

Plate 8.2 Eosinophil adherence to the cuticle of a nematode (*Trichinella spiralis*). The cell is closely adherent to the cuticle (C) and large secretion vacuoles (V) are present as a result of fusion of the characteristic granules (G). This stage is followed by the release of granule material onto the surface of the cuticle. (Photograph by courtesy of Dr D.J. McLaren.)

responses. In such hosts microfilaraemia established by transplantation of adult *D. viteae* continued for at least 182 days, whereas in normal mice the numbers of microfilariae fell rapidly and the blood became negative within 80 days (Fig. 8.7). It is interesting that there was no difference in adult worm survival between the two strains of mice, showing that immunity expressed in terms of duration of microfilaraemia was acting specifically against the survival of the larvae.

The detailed interaction between parasite, antibody and effector cells has been most fully described using *D. viteae* in rats. The Ig primarily involved in this system is IgE, acting upon the cells themselves and not functioning as an opsonizing agent, i.e. cell adherence is dependent upon the initial binding of IgE to the cell membrane rather than to the worm's cuticle. Complement-mediated adherence is also excluded in this system, there being no evidence of complement activation on the surface of newly-released microfilariae. Cell adherence, in the presence of immune serum, was evident within 1 hour. By 16 hours some 90% of larvae were heavily coated with cells and apparently dead. The first cell type to adhere was the eosinophil, making close contact with the cuticle and degranulating onto the surface of the larvae. Subsequently the layer of material released from the eosinophils lifted away and macrophages adhered in large numbers, actively phagocytosing dead cells. Macrophage adherence was followed by spreading over the cuticular surface and release of lysosomal material. At this stage the cuticle showed visible damage and there was lysis of internal tissues (Plate 8.3).

An interesting and important aspect of this study was that antibodies capable of

Table 8.3 Trapping and damage of serum-sensitized microfilaria larvae of *Dipetalonema viteae* when contained within micropore chambers (3 μm pore size) and implanted into normal hamsters. (Data from Weiss & Tanner, 1979, *Tropenmedizin Parasitologie*, **30**, 73.)

Serum used	% larvae trapped	Motility of larvae	No. of cells adherent/larva
Normal	0	Active	0
Immune	70–100	Immobile	>20
Immune (ME)	>5	Active	1–9
Immune I	80–100	Immobile	>20
Immune II	>5	Active	1–9

Chambers were recovered after 18 h in the host. (ME) = serum treated with 2-mercaptoethanol to detroy IgM. I/II = 1st (IgM enriched) and 2nd (IgM depleted) peaks obtained by fractionation of serum on Sephadex G200.

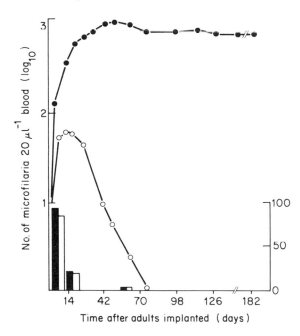

Fig. 8.7 Duration of microfilaraemia and adult worm survival in CBA/n and CBA/H mice given adult *Dipetalonema viteae* by subcutaneous implantation. No. of microfilaria: ● CBA/n, ○ CBA/H; % survival of adults: ■ CBA/n, □ CBA/H. (Redrawn from Thompson *et al.*, 1979, *Journal of Parasitology*, **65**, 966.)

mediating adherence appeared only after rats became amicrofilaraemic. While microfilaria were present in the blood no *in vitro* adherence or killing could be demonstrated. This observation is in line with a great deal of evidence from infections in man and supports the concept that anti-microfilarial responses may be an important component of human protective immunity. One puzzle is why it takes a comparatively long time for such immunity to be manifested. It is well documented

128

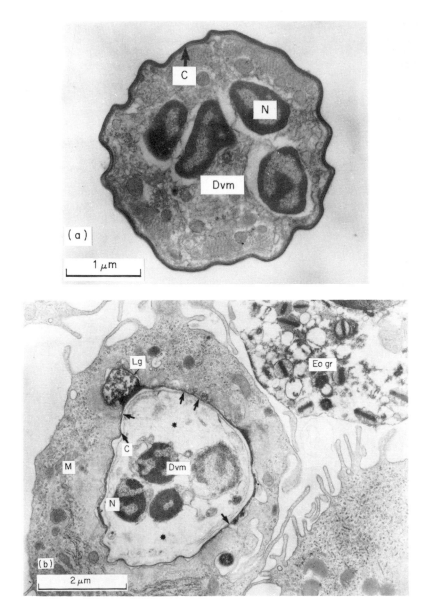

Plate 8.3 Antibody-dependent, cell-mediated destruction of microfilaria. (a) TEM of intact microfilaria of *Dipetalonema viteae* (Dvm) after 16h culture in the presence of normal rat serum and peritoneal exudate cells. The cuticle (C) is unbroken and the nucleus (N) is undamaged. (b) TEM of degenerating microfilaria of *D. viteae* (Dvm) after 16 hours culture in the presence of immune rat serum and peritoneal exudate cells. The parasite is enveloped by a macrophage (M) and lysosome-like granules (Lg) are being released on to the cuticle (C), which shows focal damage (arrows). The internal structure of the microfilaria has been lost, although nuclei (N) are still recognizable. Eo gr = granules of adjacent eosinophil. (Photographs from Haque et al., 1981, *Journal of Immunology*, **127**, 716, by permission of the author and publishers.)

that filarial infections are associated with pronounced immunosuppression and this may be one contributory factor. Another may be the fact that certain microfilariae appear to acquire host components upon their surface. The surface-labelling patterns of newly-released larvae differ from those of older larvae and there is evidence for the presence of host serum albumin on the cuticle. This may possibly act as a form of disguise, rendering the larvae both less immunogenic and less susceptible.

8.2.3   Responses against Infective Larvae and Adults of Filarial Worms

The emphasis placed upon responses against the microfilariae should not be taken to mean that there is no effective resistance against other stages in the life cycle of filarial worms. Epidemiological studies in endemic areas show that virtually all individuals will be exposed to the bites of infected vectors, yet many never develop patent infections. Some of these individuals also never show any clinical evidence of infection, even though they may be positive on immunodiagnosis. This may reflect a resistance that is effective against the infective larvae or subsequent pre-adult stages and which prevents the development of sexually-mature worms. Other individuals, though parasitologically negative, do have clinical symptoms and suffer from acute filariasis, having recurrent fevers and inflammation of the lymph nodes. This again may indicate a resistance that operates against initial stages of infection or against adult worms, preventing reproduction from taking place.

Direct evidence for immunity against infective larvae and pre-adults is difficult to obtain, despite the fact that it is relatively easy to demonstrate anti-L_3 antibodies in infected hosts. In the hamster–*D. viteae* system, for example, it appears that secondary and tertiary infections, given to animals that have become amicro-filaraemic after initial infection, develop uninterruptedly but fail to reproduce. In contrast, in the abnormal mouse host, evidence for specific anti-infective larval immunity has been obtained using larvae implanted in micropore chambers. Cats that have become amicrofilaraemic after infection with *B. pahangi* are resistant to challenge and third-stage larvae are killed before they enter the host's lymphatics. The immunogenicity of the infective stage is also confirmed by the demonstration (in certain systems) that irradiated larvae can be used to vaccinate against infection. This has been achieved with *B. malayi* in monkeys, *B. pahangi* in cats and dogs, *Dirofilaria immitis* in dogs and *L. carinii* in rats, though to variable degrees in each system.

It is reasonable to assume that immunity against the early stages of infection is achieved through various forms of ADCC, mediated by antibodies directed against surface antigens. Antibodies with larval specificity are frequently present, but not always correlated with immune status. An intriguing aspect of immunity against larvae and developmental stages is its strict thymus dependency and the manner in which this is expressed. Although mice are abnormal hosts for *B. pahangi*, it is possible to establish patent infections by injection of larvae into thymus-deficient (nude) or thymus-deprived mice. Whether the susceptibility is entirely due to an inability to produce T-dependent antibodies or reflects the absence of other forms of T cell-mediated response has yet to be clarified.

Circumstantial evidence in man suggests that immunity can operate against the adult worm stage and this is reinforced by many laboratory observations. The ways in which anti-adult immunity is expressed vary considerably between different laboratory models. In some, for example *D. viteae* in the rat, adult worms die long before microfilariae are cleared from the bloodstream. In others the host becomes amicrofilaraemic even though the adult worms remain alive. This situation occurs during infections with *D. viteae* in hamsters and it has been shown that the disappearance of microfilariae from the circulation (latency of infection) is in part due a failure of the adult female worms to liberate larvae. The immune basis for this phenomenon can be demonstrated in a variety of ways (Fig. 8.8). Latency can be induced by passive transfer of immune serum and by vaccination with worm antigen. The inhibitory action of serum is also evident against female worms maintained *in vitro*. Latent females resume microfilarial release when the host is immune suppressed or when transplanted from latent into naive hosts. It is not certain precisely what serum factor is responsible for latency. It is known to be heat labile, but it has not been identified with a particular isotype of Ig. Equally it is not known how this factor exerts its effects, although a neuropharmacological action upon the mechanisms of larval release cannot be excluded.

Antibodies against adult worm antigens are readily detectable in infected hosts, but their presence is not necessarily correlated with resistance to infection. Indeed many antibodies have specificity for antigens present internally in the worms, and these would not become available to the host until after the death of the worms.

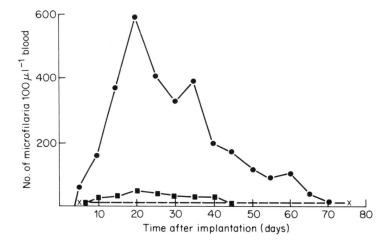

Fig. 8.8 Influence of immunity upon microfilaraemia in hamsters infected by implantation of adult *Dipetalonema viteae*. ●————● normal hamsters given 5 worms from 90-day infected (latent) donor; ■————■ normal hamsters given 5 worms from 90-day infected (latent) donor and 3 ml of immune serum; ✗————✗ latent hamsters given 5 worms from 90-day infected (latent) donor. (Data from Haque *et al.*, 1978, *Parasitology*, **76**, 61.)

8.3   Hypersensitivity and Immunopathology

The intimate and prolonged contact between filarial nematodes and the tissues of the host leads to the generation of a wide spectrum of immune responses. Although some of these are beneficial, in that they help to limit the activity or the survival of the infection, many are quite irrelevant to the well-being of the worm. A proportion of these irrelevant responses may actually be harmful to the host and contribute to the development of pathological reactions, but immunopathology may also be linked to the host-protective responses. Indeed, in the lymphatic filariases there is good evidence that the most severe pathological reactions, such as elephantiasis, are associated with the development of some degree of immunity.

Filarial infections in general are associated with high levels of reaginic antibody and pronounced eosinophilia, and there is little doubt that immediate hypersensitivity reactions are a major cause of filarial pathology. A severe consequence of infection is tropical pulmonary eosinophilia (TPE) where the patient suffers from asthmatic symptoms and interstitial lung disease. Although the precise causes are uncertain, TPE is believed to result from exaggerated immune responses against the microfilariae of species such as *W. bancrofti* and *B. malayi*. Patients with TPE show very high anti-filarial antibody titres, high total IgE and abnormally high eosinophil counts. It is possible that microfilaria are cleared from the circulation and destroyed in the lungs by ADCC reactions, with resultant cellular infiltration around trapped larvae. This mode of antigen presentation is known in experimental models to lead to eosinophilia and may also potentiate reaginic responses.

Immediate hypersensitivity responses may also play an important role in the intense itching and the development of the pathological skin changes associated with chronic *Onchocerca* infection. Among the significant histological findings are infiltrations by mast cells, eosinophils, lymphocytes, plasma cells and macrophages. These may be initiated by antibody reacting with free antigen released from microfilariae. The presence of mast cells, reaginic antibody and worm antigen clearly provides the basis for exaggerated skin reactivity. Immediate responses may also accompany the formation of the nodules around adult worms, as these are often surrounded by eosinophils (Plate 8.4).

Treatment of filarial infections, particularly onchocerciasis, with the drug diethylcarbamazine (DEC) can elicit particularly powerful hypersensitivity responses known as the Mazzotti reactions. The reaction is triggered by the sudden presentation of massive amounts of microfilarial antigen, released by the death of the larvae or

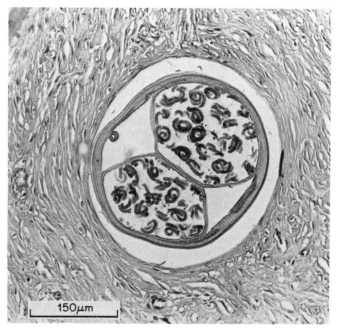

Plate 8.4 Response to adult *Onchocerca volvulus* in man. The section shown the fibrous connective tissue nodule that forms around the adult worms. Within the worm can be seen the uteri containing microfilaria larvae.

made available by a drug-induced 'unmasking' of surface antigens. DEC also appears to enhance the host's ADCC response against the larvae.

Delayed type hypersensitivity reactions (DTH) are also involved in filarial pathology and may contribute to the development of obstructive lesions around dead or dying worms in lymphatic filariases.

Patients with elephantiasis show greater lymphocyte responsiveness to adult worm antigens than do patients with other symptoms. Dermal changes caused by *O. volvulus* may also involve DTH in some circumstances (possibly in the 'sowdah' form of the disease), but there is often an inverse relationship between the numbers of microfilariae present in the skin and the degree of DTH measurable by antigen injection or by lymphocyte proliferation.

The exaggerated antibody responses associated with filarial infections and the large amounts of antigen available obviously predispose to the formation of immune complexes. There is indeed evidence for the presence of such complexes, but their role in pathogenesis is far from clear. Deposition of complexes may initiate Arthus reactions in infected lymphatics and infected skin, and may be a contributory factor in the development of eye lesions in onchocerciasis. Although the latter have been well described the causes underlying their formation are poorly understood, although responses against microfilarial antigens must play the major role.

As with other chronic parasite infections, filariasis is often accompanied by a degree of immune suppression. Several studies have shown a reduced reactivity to parasite antigens in human patients, using cell-mediated responses as the test system, but the immune suppression appears to be specific, in that responses to unrelated antigens are not impaired (Fig. 8.9). A variety of animals models have been used to explore this phenomenon and in some, as in man, suppressor T cell have been identified. Mitogen responsiveness may also be suppressed in rodent infections, but the significance of this observation, as far as man is concerned, is uncertain. Immune suppression is greatest when the host is microfilaraemic and least when microfilariae have been cleared from the blood stream. This implies either that microfilariae are the source of antigens or other factors which lead to suppression, or that reversal of suppressive influences allows the host to remove microfilarial stages.

Despite the suppression of immune responsiveness that filarial infections induce there is little evidence for increased host susceptibility to other pathogens. Immune suppression may well be a strategy that the parasite uses to promote its own survival, but it may be 'permitted' by the host because, by reducing anti-parasite responses, it reduces the degree of pathology that infection elicits. The chronic infections that characterize this group of worms may therefore reflect a balanced relationship that has arisen by evolutionary adaptation. Clearly the host would be better off without the parasite, but the cost of achieving total immunity may not be worthwhile.

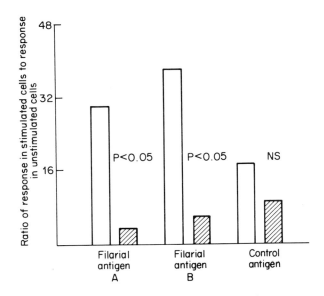

Fig. 8.9 Depression of lymphocyte responsiveness in children infected with *Wuchereria bancrofti*. Peripheral blood lymphocytes were cultured *in vitro* with either *Brugia malayi* antigen (A), *Dirofilaria immitis* antigen (B) or tuberculin antigen or streptococcal antigen (control). Responsiveness was measured by uptake of ^{3}H thymidine. ☐ children exposed but not microfilaraemic; ▨ children with microfilaraemia. (Redrawn from Ottesen *et al.*, 1977, *Immunology*, **33**, 413.)

9

Ectoparasitic Arthropods

Immunity at the Surface of the Body

Terrestrial vertebrates act as hosts for a variety of ectoparasitic arthropods. Infestation with such parasites may give rise to pathological symptoms, through damage to dermal tissues or systemic effects, but of far greater significance is the transmission of infectious organisms, from viruses to helminths, for which arthropods act as vectors. As a way of life, ectoparasitism is harder to categorize than endoparasitism. In the latter the host provides the total environment, contact is intimate and prolonged, and the parasite exhibits complete metabolic dependency. In the former the parasite may make only intermittent contact for the purposes of feeding, and spend long periods away from the host. As with all biological phenomena, however, there is a wide spectrum of associations covered by the term ectoparasitism and this is reflected both in the duration and the intimacy of host contact. In mammals, for example, the extremes can be illustrated by the scabies mite (*Sarcoptes scabei*), which spends its whole life upon the host and burrows into the skin, and by the mosquito, in which only the female is parasitic, making sporadic host contact in order to feed briefly before egg laying.

9.1   Responses to Feeding

With all ectoparasites, the point of host contact is the skin and it is through this organ that protective responses are initiated. If the parasite is accessible, protection may be achieved through the entirely non-specific mechanisms of scratching or grooming. Immune responses, particularly immediate hypersensitivity reactions, may enhance this non-specific protection by making the host more aware of the presence of the parasite. Where the parasite is less accessible, less easily dislodged, or where the host is less able to groom, then immune responses with a direct, anti-parasite effect may play an important role in protection.

The skin is well equipped to make protective responses, its extensive vascularization providing ready access for humoral and cellular effectors. In addition, the resident amine-containing cells form a sentinel population capable of rapid reaction to tissue damage and, by their degranulation, allowing enhanced infiltration of other cell populations. There is a characteristic population of dendritic, antigen-presenting cells, the Langerhans cells, which are ideally situated for processing antigens presented during the feeding of the parasite. All ectoparasites introduce saliva into the wound made by their mouthparts and in many cases this contains anticoagulant factors which prevent blood from clotting. The proteins present in saliva are potent immunogens and elicit strong immune responses, frequently hypersensitive in nature. The effect of these responses upon the parasite is of course related to the duration of feeding. If this is less than the time necessary for the development of the response then the parasite feeds and escapes unscathed. With longer feeding times the response generated has the opportunity to affect the parasite. The nature of skin-based protective responses have been investigated most thoroughly in host–parasite associations involving ticks.

9.2 Immune Responses to Ticks

Ticks belong to a large group of the arachnid arthropods, the Acarina. They are distinguished from the closely-related mites by their larger size and by their host relationships. All are parasitic and all are blood feeders throughout their development. Many transmit serious pathogens to man and to domestic animals and are major pests, particularly in countries with warm climates (Table 9.1).

Table 9.1 Pathogens and diseases transmitted to man and domestic animals by ticks.

Genus	Pathogen	Disease
Soft ticks		
Ornithodorus	Spirochaetes	Relapsing fever
Hard ticks		
Amblyomma	Rickettsias	Spotted fever
	Bacteria	Tularaemia
Boophilus	Protozoa (Babesia)	Piroplasmosis
Dermacentor	Viruses	Encephalomyelitis
	Rickettsias	Spotted fever
	Bacteria	Tularaemia
	Protozoa (Babesia)	Piroplasmosis
Haemaphysalis	Rickettsias	Spotted fever
	Bacteria	Tularaemia
	Protozoa (Babesia)	Piroplasmosis
Hyalomma	Rickettsias	Rickettsiosis
	Protozoa (Theileria)	East Coast fever
Ixodes	Viruses	Encephalomyelitis
	Rickettsias	Tick typhus
	Protozoa (Babesia)	Piroplasmosis
Rhipicephalus	Viruses	Encephalomyelitis
	Spirochaetes	Tick typhus
	Protozoa (Babesia, Theileria)	Piroplasmosis East Coast fever

Ticks show a variety of host-contact patterns during their life cycles. In some species each developmental stage feeds upon the same host individual, in others two or three individuals are used, with the ticks leaving the host when replete in order to moult. In three host ticks a different individual is used by each stage in the cycle, i.e. larva, nymph and adult, and one blood meal is taken on each host. (These patterns characterize the hard (ixodiid) ticks, soft (argasid) ticks feed more frequently.) The feeding of hard ticks is a lengthy process and may take several days. The mouthparts are adapted for cutting into the skin and for taking up blood. Feeding is preceded by production of saliva and of a cement-like material which serves to hold the mouthparts firmly in the skin (Plate 9.1). The antigenic material contained within these secretions persists in the skin for several days after feeding and can be

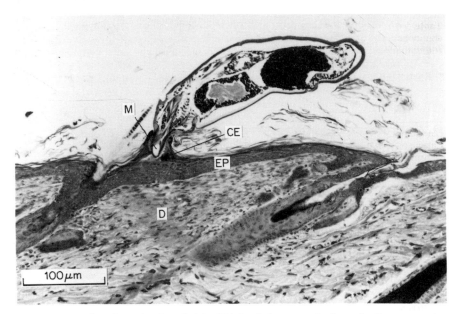

Plate 9.1 Section through a larval tick, *Rhipicephalus appendiculatus*, feeding on a naive guinea pig 12–24 hours after attachment. The mouthparts (M), anchored by cement (CE) are superficial in the epidermis (EP) and do not penetrate into the dermis (D). (Photograph by courtesy of Dr S.J. Brown.)

identified, by fluorescent labelling, on the surface of the Langerhans cells. Even on naive hosts tick bites lead to pronounced inflammatory responses, but these do not prevent engorgement. In the immune host the reaction to biting is rapid and may prevent feeding completely. Failure to feed quickly causes the death of the tick, from the combined effects of starvation and desiccation.

Immunity to ixodiid ticks was first described as long ago as 1939 by Trager, who found that larval stages of *Dermacentor variabilis* were completely unable to feed upon guinea-pigs that had been exposed to repeated experimental infestations. It has also been known for many years, initially from empirical field observations, that there is acquired resistance to ticks in cattle, some individuals and some breeds developing greater immunity than others. In recent years guinea-pig models of tick immunity have been intensively studied (Table 9.2). The kinetics of the response have been described in detail and the underlying mechanisms have been very fully analysed. Immunity is easily assessed in this system and is usually measured from the percentage of ticks which successfully complete their feeding and become fully engorged (Table 9.3).

Table 9.2 Species of ticks used in experimental studies of immunity in the guinea-pig host.

Amblyomma americanum	*I. holocyclus*
Dermacentor andersoni	*Rhipicephalus*
D. variabilis	*appendiculatus*
Ixodes dammini	*R. sanguineus*

Table 9.3 Effect of immunity established by initial infestation upon development of challenges with tick larvae in guinea-pigs. (Data from Brown & Askenase, 1981, *Journal of Immunology*, **127**, 2163.)

	Amblyomma		Rhipicephalus	
	% recovery of ticks	Weight of ticks (mg)	% recovery of ticks	Weight of ticks (mg)
Larvae on control hosts	80	0.95	73	0.28
Larvae on immune hosts	34	0.58	28	0.20
% rejection of larvae	58	–	62	–
% reduction in weight	–	39	–	29

9.3 Analysis of Immunity

Many studies, using a variety of ixodiid ticks, have shown that an effective and long-lasting immunity develops extremely rapidly, being apparent within a week of initial infection. On immune hosts ticks fail to engorge, show impaired moulting, and may die from desiccation within 24 hours. The immune response to infestation is remarkably sensitive and experiments have shown that guinea-pigs exposed to one mature female tick for more than 48 hours develop nearly complete immunity against a subsequent challenge with 200 larvae. As this indicates, immunity is not stage-specific; all stages in the life cycle can immunize against larvae, and larvae immunize against nymphs.

Immunity is not a local phenomenon and once elicited will operate effectively at sites remote from the original feeding area. Transfer of immunity can be achieved using either immune serum or immune lymphocytes and very high levels of protection (up to 95%) have been conferred on recipients with as little as 0.5 ml of serum (Table 9.4). The degree of immunity that can be transferred varies between systems, depending upon the species of tick and the strain of Guinea-pig, and this may reflect differences in the ways in which effective responses are generated.

Table 9.4 Transfer of immunity to *Rhipicephalus appendiculatus* in Guinea-pigs given transfers of immune sera, or immune peritoneal exudate cells (PEC) from donors exposed to larval infestations. (Data from Askenase *et al.*, 1982, *Immunology*, **45**, 501.)

		% reduction in challenge larvae recovered compared with non-immune hosts
Immune sera		
(vol./recipient)	2 ml	97
	1 ml	92
	0.5 ml	76
	0.25 ml	8
Control* serum	2 ml	12
Immune PEC		
(no./recipient)	2×10^8	87
Control* PEC	2×10^8	1

*Control sera and cells taken from guinea pigs immunized against *Trichinella spiralis*.

9.3.1   Cellular Basis of Immunity

The distinctive features of the local skin reactions to ticks on an immune host are a massive infiltration of basophils at the dermal–epidermal junction and a smaller, though still pronounced, infiltrate of eosinophils (Fig. 9.1). Mononuclear cells are an

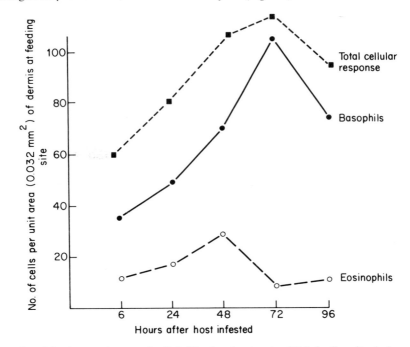

Fig. 9.1   Numbers and types of cells infiltrating the dermis of tick feeding sites in immune guinea pigs infected with *Rhipicephalus appendiculatus*. (Data from Brown *et al.*, 1983, *Experimental Parasitology*, **55**, 111.)

important constituent in the response against certain species. Infiltration is correlated with rises in the number of basophils and eosinophils circulating in the peripheral blood. It was recognized several years ago that the reactions have the characteristics of a cutaneous basophil hypersensitivity (CBH) response and there is now a great deal of circumstantial evidence that basophils play a key role in resistance. Rejection of challenge infections is correlated with the arrival and degranulation of these cells and is directly related to the host's ability to mount a CBH response. Resistance is blocked by treatment with cytostatic immunosuppressive agents such as cyclophosphamide and methotrexate and can be specifically inhibited by treatment with an anti-basophil serum.

Although the mechanisms through which resistance is expressed is closely associated with degranulation of basophils, and thus the release of a variety of inflammatory mediators, it is not known whether these mediators act directly against the tick or act via alterations in the environment of the immediate feeding area. Basophils have also been seen within the intestines of ticks fed on immune hosts, and it is possible that release of mediators within the tick itself could lead to damage and death. However, similar basophil uptake has been described in soft ticks and these appear to survive unimpaired. Alterations of the tissues at the feeding site would

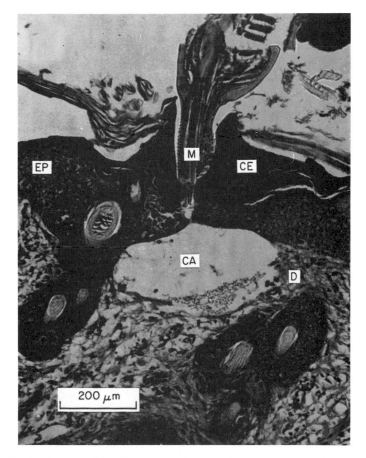

Plate 9.2 Section through head of a nymphal tick, *Amblyomma americana*, feeding on a naive guinea pig 12 hours after attachment. The mouthparts (M), anchored by cement (CE) have penetrated through the epidermis (EP) into the dermis (D). Feeding activity has resulted in the formation of a cavity (CA) into which host cells will infiltrate. (Photograph from Brown & Knapp, 1980, *Experimental Parasitology*, **49**, 188, by permission of the authors and publishers.)

change the quantity and quality of blood available, and this would be reflected in both reduced uptake and deficient metabolism. A major component of basophil granules is histamine and it may be significant that in cattle, where basophils also predominate in the dermal response to infestation, injection of histamine directly into feeding sites causes ticks to detach; injection of anti-histamines prolongs feeding and survival. In addition it has been shown that factors which inactivate histamine have been identified in tick feeding secretions.

Although basophils form a major element in the infiltrating cell population there is evidence that an important component of resistance is basophil-mediated chemotactic recruitment of eosinophils, which also accumulate at feeding sites. Treatment of the host with an anti-basophil serum, though it has no effect on eosinophil numbers in the blood or bone marrow, significantly reduces the number of eosinophils present at the feeding site. Treatment with an anti-eosinophil serum has

Table 9.5 Effect of treating immune Guinea-pigs with rabbit anti-basophil (ABS) or anti-eosinophil (AES) sera on their resistance to challenge with larvae of *Amblyomma americanum* and the numbers of cells present at the tick feeding sites. (Data from Brown & Askenase, 1983, *Federation Proceedings*, **42**, 1744.)

Host Group	Treatment	% rejection of challenge	Mean numbers of cells at feeding site (0.032 mm^{-2})		
			Basophils	Eosinophils	Mononuclear
Control	Nil, SAL or NRS*	–	23	12	25
Immune	Nil or SAL*	48	81	87	54
Immune	NRS	47	67	91	58
Immune	AES	23	58	19	72
Immune	ABS	7	1	34	93

*Control treatments with nothing (Nil), saline (SAL) or normal rabbit serum (NRS).

no effect on numbers of basophils but nevertheless significantly impairs resistance (Table 9.5). As has already been discussed, in the context of resistance against schistosome infections, eosinophils release a variety of factors (e.g. peroxidases, major basic protein) which are capable of damaging and killing parasites. Equally, their cytotoxic efficiency is increased in the presence of mediators (e.g. ECF–A tetrapeptides) released by amine-containing cells, and there is evidence that eosinophil peroxidases may have greater activity when bound to basophil granules. Resistance to ticks is therefore achieved by a cooperative interaction between basophils and eosinophils, the former playing a major role in initiating and focussing cellular infiltration at the feeding site.

The generation of the basophil response may involve at least three distinct mechanisms, mediated through T cells, antibody or complement components. Evidence for these mechanisms is summarized as follows.

1. Adoptive transfer of immunity against ticks can be achieved using suspensions of lymphocytes or peritoneal exudate cells. It is assumed, from the data available from detailed studies on CBH responses to defined antigens, that the effective cells are T lymphocytes. Such cells liberate lymphokines capable of attracting basophils to sites of antigen deposition and may also contribute to basophil degranulation, thus enhancing further cell recruitment by increasing vascular and tissue permeability and releasing chemotactic factors.

2. The immunoglobulins associated with passive transfer of resistance to ticks in guinea-pigs have been identified as belonging to the IgG_1 isotype, a class known to be involved in CBH responses against other antigens. Although the precise role of the IgG_1 is uncertain, it has been suggested that it contributes, via amine-cell degranulation, to a cascade reaction that again facilitates cell recruitment through chemotaxis and increased permeability.

3. Fluorescent-labelling studies have shown the presence of antigen–antibody complexes at the dermal–epidermal junctions near feeding ticks. Complement is activated by such complexes and particular activation products, e.g. C5a, are known to attract basophil cells. Certainly the degree of basophil infiltration is reduced when the host is depleted of complement.

9.3.2 Tick Antigens and Immunity

The fact that ectoparasties have close physiological contact with the host only when feeding makes it obvious that the source of immunogens must be the secretions injected into the host during the process. Not only can tick antigens be identified in the tissues underlying the feeding site, but it has been well established that crude extracts of ticks can be used to stimulate an effective immunity (Table 9.6). Immunization is effective even in the absence of adjuvant. There is good evidence for cross-reactivity between antigens released by different species of ticks, and this is reflected in cross-resistance, both in hosts actively immunized by infection and in animals passively immunized with serum. These observations augur well for the use of controlled induction of resistance as a means of tick control in the field. There are abundant data to show that resistant cattle are more productive in areas where ticks are endemic and also that, as a result of their tick resistance, they suffer less from the diseases which ticks transmit. However, there is obviously a complex inter-relationship between host, tick and infectious organism. This has been well illustrated by studies upon cattle infected with *Babesia bovis*, an intracellular protozoan transmitted by the tick *Boophilus microplus*. *B. bovis*, like many protozoans, can exert a profound immunosuppressive effect upon the host. Cattle suppressed by infection show much less resistance to the vector tick and, in consequence, aquire much heavier infestations. By achieving this, of course, the protozoan optimizes its

Table 9.6 Immunization of calves against infestation with *Dermacentor andersoni* by prior injection of tick homogenate. Each calf received 30 ♂ and 100 ♀ ticks 3 days after the third injection of 67 mg homogenate protein and ticks were removed 10 days later when engorgement should have been completed. (Data from Allen & Humphreys, 1979, *Nature*, **280**, 491.)

	Ticks recovered				Total egg production ($\times 10^{-3}$)
Group	Mean no.	Mean weight	No. of dead part-fed ♀	No. of ♀ laying eggs	
Control	107	24g	12	50	164
Immunized	97	4g	44	15	28

own survival and dispersal. This complexity of host-parasite relationships in the field places severe constraints upon the application of immunologically-based strategies for control. At the same time it also illustrates the substantial benefits to be gained by the implementation of really effective immunization regimes.

10

Immunological Control of Parasitic Infections

An ultimate objective for immunoparasitologists is the production of vaccines that will protect man and domestic animals against the debilitating effects of parasitic infections. It has to be confessed, however, that to date, realization of this objective in practical terms has met with very limited success. Few vaccines have ever reached the stage of commercial prodution and only two, those against lungworm and *Babesia* infections in cattle, are presently marketed on a large scale. The reasons for such limited success are multiple and include:

(*i*)   lack of knowledge of the mechanisms involved in protective immune responses,
(*ii*) lack of knowledge of the antigens that elicit protective immune responses,
(*iii*) inability to produce antigenic material in sufficient quantity,
(*iv*) failure to vaccinate effectively under field conditions,
(*v*)   failure to satisfy commercial and user requirements.

10.1 Vaccination against Lungworms in Cattle

It is instructive to consider the success of the lungworm vaccine in the light of these difficulties. Lungworms, *Dictyocaulus* spp., are nematodes parasitic in cattle, sheep and other ruminants. The species against which the vaccine is protective, *D. viviparus*, affects cattle and can give rise to severe epidemics of respiratory disease. In Britain lungworm disease – 'Husk' – was worst along the West coast, where the milder, wetter climate favoured the survival of the infective larval stages on pasture (Fig. 10.1). In bad years infections caused the deaths of thousands of animals and an economic loss of millions of pounds. Animals which survived the disease become highly resistant to reinfection, but the responses underlying this resistance and the antigens which elicit these responses are not identified. The pathogenic stages of the life cycle are the adult worms, which live in the bronchioles of the lungs and induce severe inflammatory responses (Plate 10.1). The larval stages, which migrate from the intestine to the lungs, are relatively harmless.

Study of the developmental stages of *D. viviparus* and of immunity engendered by infection were facilitated by the fact that the parasite can be readily established in a laboratory host, the guinea-pig, and can be maintained easily from the larvae passed by infected calves. Experimental studies showed that the stage which elicited

144

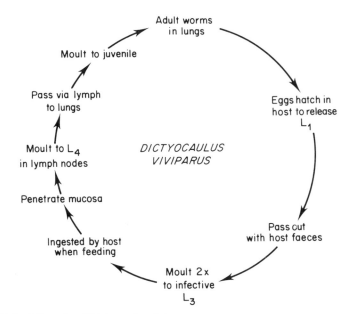

Fig. 10.1 Life cycle of *Dictyocaulus viviparus*.

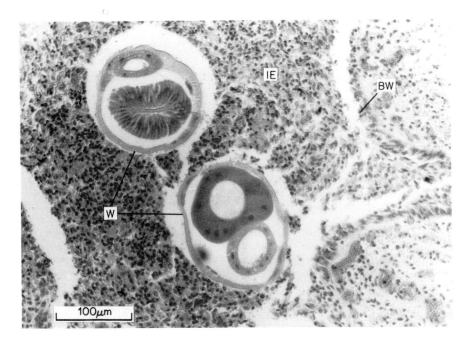

Plate 10.1 Response to the lungworm *Dictyocaulus viviparus* in an infected calf. The section was made from tissue taken from a calf killed by infection. The lumen of the bronchiole is filled with an inflammatory exudate (IE) surrounding adult worms (W). BW = bronchiole wall.

immunity, and which was affected by the immune response, was the fourth larval stage, i.e. the stage preceding development of the pathogenic adult worms. This was a most fortuitous and most important finding, as it meant that it became possible to think in terms of artificially inducing immunity, but avoiding pathology, by restricting the development of the worm. The method of choice for achieving this restriction was that of radiation-induced attenuation. The guinea-pig model was used to develop a suitable immunization protocol using infective third-stage larvae irradiated at 40 krad. At this level, larvae develop only to the fourth stage and then die. It was found possible to stimulate high levels (> 90%) of immunity by giving two doses, each of

Table 10.1 A   Immunity to challenge with *Dictyocaulus viviparus* in guinea-pigs immunized by infection with 2 × 5000 40 k rad irradiated larvae (source as below).

Day after challenge	No. of larvae recovered from lungs after challenge with normal larvae	
	Control hosts	Immunized hosts
2	140	37
4	69	9
6	136	0
8	375	0

Table 10.1 B   Comparison of immunization with normal or irradiated larvae. (Data from Poynter *et al.*, 1960, *Veterinary Record*, **72**, 1078.)

Day after challenge	Mean larval recovery		
	Control hosts	Immunized hosts	
		Irradiated larvae	Normal larvae
10	331	0.4	1.0

1000 irradiated larvae, at an interval of 3 to 4 weeks (Table 10.1). The protocol worked equally well with cattle, thus providing the basis for development of the vaccine on a commercial scale. Four factors greatly influenced the success of the commercial venture:

(*i*) supplies of larvae were readily available from faeces of infected calves and infective third-stage larvae for irradiation were easily cultured,

(*ii*) infection, and therefore administration of the vaccine, were via the oral route and so there were no overriding problems with sterility of the product,

(*iii*) at the time that the vaccine was under development there were no satisfactory alternative treatments, chemotherapy being relatively inefficient,

(*iv*) the vaccine could be administered by the farmer.

10.2   Vaccination against Hookworms in Dogs

The success of the lungworm vaccine may be contrasted with the commercial failure of the vaccine developed for the control of hookworm (*Ancylostoma caninum*) infections in dogs, an important veterinary problem in the U.S.A. The hookworm vaccine was also based upon the use of irradiation-attenuated infective larvae, but in this case infection and vaccine administration were parenteral. Injection of the vaccine required a degree of sterility that was initially difficult to achieve with organisms necessarily cultured from faecal material. This difficulty was overcome and the vaccine was marketed widely. It was highly effective in preventing hookworm disease, but, like lungworm vaccine, did not completely prevent infection. The presence of hookworm eggs in the faeces of vaccinated dogs led to suspicions of vaccine failure, even though no overt disease developed. Effective anthelmintic chemotherapy was readily available and many veterinarians, faced with the choice of giving the vaccine or a drug, preferred the latter. Ultimately the vaccine was withdrawn.

10.3   Field Failures of Experimental Vaccines

Several promising vaccines have never reached the stage of commercial production despite giving high levels of protection in experimental trials under controlled conditions. One good example of this situation, again drawn from nematode infections of veterinary significance, concerns the irradiation-attenuated vaccine devised to protect against *Haemonchus contortus* in sheep. In trials, using lambs of 7 to 8 months and mature sheep, the vaccine was highly effective, reducing worm burdens from challenge infections by as much as 98%. In the field, however, it proved difficult if not impossible to confer any protection upon young lambs, the age-group most at risk, or older sheep that had acquired infection as young lambs. The unresponsiveness of young lambs to *H. contortus* and the 'tolerance' of older infected animals remain unexplained, but are major obstacles to successful vaccination.

Several other cases can be cited of experimental vaccines which work well under laboratory conditions, but which cannot be scaled up for field use because of limited amounts of antigen, or which are valueless in the field because of limitations imposed by the specificity of protection they stimulate. It is perfectly possible, for example, to raise virtually complete immunity to challenge with specific VATs of trypanosomes, but in the field, vaccination has to contend with the phenomenon of antigenic variation, at present an insuperable difficulty.

10.4   The Future for Anti-Parasite Vaccines

The problems encountered in the past in devising anti-parasite vaccines have engendered a rather pessimistic attitude to the possibility of ever being able to vaccinate successfully against the major parasitic diseases, but there are now some grounds for cautious optimism in this field. The incentives to devise vaccines remain as great as ever, given the serious clinical and economic problems caused by parasitic infections and by the costs involved in solutions based upon improvements in hygiene, sanitation or environmental control. Equally, the chronic nature of many infections acquired early in life, e.g. schistosomiasis and filariasis, places a high premium on protecting the vulnerable young. Many of the major diseases of man are vector-transmitted and there are enormous problems in vector control, ranging from the difficulties of providing adequate financial support for control measures and of obtaining national and international cooperation for their implementation, to insecticide resistance and environmental pollution. These problems strengthen the case for preventing infection of vectors rather than attempting to eliminate vector populations. One way of achieving this would be to mount intensive programmes of chemotherapy, but these are often difficult to implement and, in many cases, safe self-administered drugs are either not available or are too expensive.

All of these factors point irresistably to the need for vaccines capable of giving long-lasting protection. Progress towards this ideal can be considered under the five headings given above (page 143) and then discussed in relation to specific infections.

10.4.1 The Mechanisms Involved in Protective Immune Responses

As earlier chapters have demonstrated, there has been substantial progress in understanding some of the fundamental immunological interactions between hosts and parasites. In a number of infections (e.g. malaria, schistosomiasis, filariasis) it is now possible to pinpoint the parasitic stages that are vulnerable to immunological attack and to identify the effector mechanisms which operate in their destruction or removal. Such knowledge makes it possible to consider boosting specific elements of the immune response in order to enhance the effectors involved rather than simply attempt overall stimulation of the immune response. The approaches that are relevant in this context include 'antigen engineering' to selectively increase antibody production or T-cell responsiveness, and the use of non-specific immunostimulants to enhance macrophage function. An important element is the greater awareness that now exists of the immunopathological and immunomodulatory effects exerted by infections. This makes it possible to design vaccines which selectively boost host-protective immune responses and which minimize parasite-protective or host-destructive responses.

10.4.2 The Antigens which Elicit Protective Immune Responses

Progress in understanding and manipulating mechanisms of protective immunity is intimately bound up with progress in identifying 'functional' antigens, i.e. the antigens specifically involved in eliciting resistance. Knowledge of such antigens has increased substantially in recent years and is likely to grow rapidly with the use of the techniques of contemporary immunobiology and molecular biology. One example that has already been discussed is the use of surface-labelling techniques, which has revolutionized the study of protozoan and helmith surface antigens. Another is the ability to raise monoclonal antibodies by hybridoma technology (Fig. 10.2). This technique makes it possible to obtain reagents with specificity for single antigenic determinants and thus identify very precisely molecules relevant to protective immunity. Coupling of such antibodies to solid-phase carriers simplifies the task of isolating and purifying particular antigens (e.g. by affinity chromatography) in order to obtain material for detailed biochemical and immunochemical analysis. The specificity of antigen recognition that monoclonal antibodies provide also allows the screening of polypeptides produced by *in vitro* translation of parasite-derived mRNA or by DNA recombinant technology (see below) for the presence of antigens known to be expressed *in vivo*.

10.4.3 Production of Antigenic Material in Quantity

Of the many antigens presented by intact parasites, relatively few are of major significance in stimulating immunity. Therefore, even if relatively large amounts of native parasite material can be obtained and the relevant antigens identified, the yield of these antigens from any purification procedure is likely to be small. For this reason many approaches to vaccination have concentrated on the use of attenuated live organisms, and it has to be admitted that the living parasite is often considerably more immunogenic than defined fractions prepared from it. For some species (e.g. schistosomes, gastrointestinal nematodes, lungworms) it is possible to produce relatively large numbers of infective stages from experimentally-infected animals to

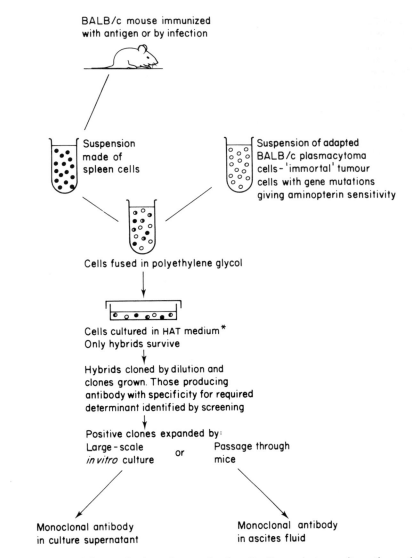

BALB/c mouse immunized
with antigen or by infection

Suspension
made of
spleen cells

Suspension of adapted
BALB/c plasmacytoma
cells - 'immortal' tumour
cells with gene mutations
giving aminopterin sensitivity

Cells fused in polyethylene glycol

Cells cultured in HAT medium*
Only hybrids survive

Hybrids cloned by dilution and
clones grown. Those producing
antibody with specificity for required
determinant identified by screening

Positive clones expanded by:
Large - scale   or   Passage through
in vitro culture   mice

Monoclonal antibody   Monoclonal antibody
in culture supernatant   in ascites fluid

Fig. 10.2 Protocol for production of monoclonal antibodies against parasite antigens. (*
HAT medium contains *h*ypoxanthine, *a*minopterin and *t*hymidine. Plasmacytoma line cells die
because of sensitivity to aminopterin, preventing utilization of the DNA precursors. Hybrid
cells survive by virtue of the normal genes introduced from the spleen cells. Spleen cells do not
replicate.)

use in vaccine production. However, the limited life-span of these stages has
presented a major problem. Development of successful cryopreservation techniques
has facilitated storage and stock-piling of material and this approach has been used in
the production of trial vaccines against schistosomiasis in cattle (see page 153). For
many parasites of man, such as filarial nematodes, large amounts of parasite material
cannot be produced from natural or experimental infections and alternative sources

are necessary. A partial solution lies in *in vitro* culture, and in recent years major successes in this field have been in the culture of *Plasmodium falciparum* and of bloodstream trypanosomes. Although such technical advances have made available large numbers of organisms of antigenic analysis and other immunological studies they cannot be considered as candidates for vaccine production directly. Less success has been achieved with helminths, which do not replicate as prolifically as protozoans, but some progress has been made in providing material for vaccination of sheep and cattle against infection with larval tapeworms.

A longer term approach to the question of providing sufficient amounts of material is the synthesis of parasite antigens, either chemically or by the use of recombinant DNA technology. Gene cloning, the basis of which is illustrated in Fig. 10.3, allows the expression of eukaryote genetic material in organisms such as *Escherichia coli*.

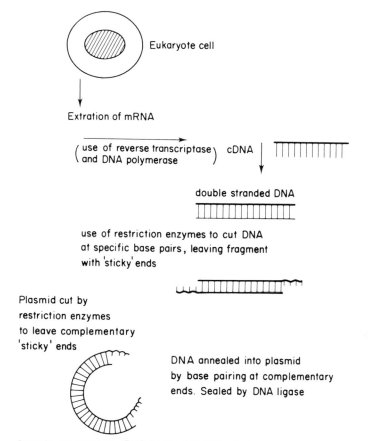

Fig. 10.3 Representation of one means of gene cloning, using mRNA to prepare cDNA and then double-stranded DNA to insert into the vector plasmid. Other ways of preparing DNA can be used, including synthesis from known sequences of the gene product concerned.

When attempting to clone the genes of ill-defined organisms such as parasites it is of course necessary to have some preliminary idea of the likely antigens and to have some means of identifying their presence, e.g. by using specific monoclonal antibodies. As will be discussed later, some progress has been made in their field and genes have already been cloned for candidate antigens of malarial and schistosome parasites.

The ability to produce specific antigen polypeptides in large amounts and with a high degree of purity will make it possible to undertake detailed analysis of their molecular structure. With this information it may then be realistic to attempt chemical or biosynthesis of specific peptide sequences in the antigen molecule and to use these, rather than the complete molecule, in attempts to immunize against infection. The rationale behind this approach (Fig. 10.4) is derived from the fact that

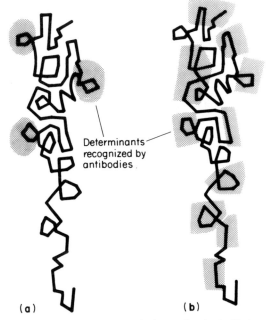

Determinants recognized by antibodies.

(a)   (b)

Fig. 10.4 Diagrammatic representation of the rationale behind synthesis of peptide sequences from target molecules for use in vaccination. (a) Antigenic determinants recognized by antibodies raised by immunization with intact molecule. (b) Antigenic determinants on intact molecule recognized by antibodies raised by immunization with synthesized peptide sequences. (Based on Lerner, 1982, *Nature*, **299**, 592.)

complex protein molecules in the native state express fewer antigenic sites than their two-dimensional structure would suggest. This is because these antigenic sites are dependent upon tertiary structural arrangements brought about by folding of the molecule. Thus immunization against the intact molecules may elicit a restricted range of antibodies with specificity for only those antigenic determinants available *in vivo*. As has been shown with several molecules, (Moloney leukaemia virus protein, chicken egg-white lysozyme, influenza virus agglutinin), however, it is possible to raise antibodies against restricted peptide sequences not 'seen' in the native molecule and to use these to interact with that molecule. In the case of the influenza agglutinin such antibodies could effectively neutralize the virus and inhibit infectivity. In parasite systems where antibody recognition of antigenic determinants is an initial step in expression of resistance through interference with behaviour (malaria merozoites and sporozoites) or through the activity of cytotoxic cells (schistosomes, filarial worms) such an approach might have considerable potential. It would also, to some extent, compensate for the inability of biosynthetic techniques to generate the carbohydrate moieties of glycoprotein antigens, where these play important roles in immunity *in vivo*.

10.4.4   Stimulation of Immunity under Field Conditions

Even allowing for the difficulties inherent in scaling-up experimental vaccines to meet field requirements, there are additional problems in the transition to field usage. Prominent among these is the requirement for vaccination to protect genetically heterogeneous populations that may be infected concurrently with other infectious organisms and be under nutritional stress. Awareness of the influence of genetic restrictions upon induction and expression of immunity has been a major development in immunoparasitology and there are now may detailed studies which have analysed the ways in which such restrictions arise. In certain cases, where low responsiveness appears linked to inadequate or delayed antibody responses, there is every possibility of presenting antigenic material in such as way that responsiveness is improved, e.g. by linking antigens to immunogenic carriers. Knowledge of immunological interactions beween concurrent infections of the immunological consequences of both protein-calorie and trace-element deficiencies has increased greatly and is beginning to provide a rational basis for corrective measures. Nevertheless, it has to be recognized that both situations impose severe limitations on the potential value of vaccination in certain conditions.

10.4.5   Commercial and User Requirements

Commercial incentives for the development of vaccines against parasitic infections remain linked to the likely profitability of such ventures. Vaccines against infections which are prevalent in developing nations offer little prospect for profitability unless there is intervention from international funding agencies. Initiatives of this kind are already in existence for the development of chemotherapeutic control and will undoubtedly be extended to the immunoprophylactic field. User requirements for vaccines pose many problems in addition to the obvious ones of reliability and safety. There are considerable logistic difficulties in making labile materials available in tropical counties, where limitations of transport and storage facilities may restrict effective distribution. There are also problems of user acceptability if adjuvant materials have to be incorporated into vaccines and if there are risks, however slight, of immunopathological side-effects. Many purified antigens lack the adjuvanticity associated with crude mixtures of parasite material or indeed with the live infection. Provision of defined antigens through recombinant technology may go some way towards providing stable, easily distributable vaccines, and progress in adjuvant development may soon solve the difficulties inherent in the use of conventional adjuvant preparations.

10.5   Progress in Development of Vaccines against Specific Infections

The previous sections have looked at future vaccines from the speculative viewpoint of 'what might be'. To bring the topic back to reality the progress made in developing vaccines against two of the major parasitic infections of man, malaria and schistosomiasis, will be briefly considered.

10.5.1   Malaria

The prevalence of malaria in tropical and subtropical regions of the world, the severity of the disease, particularly in children, and the ready transmission of infection to tourists or military personnel have long made vaccination a desirable objective. Many factors operate against the achievement of this objective, including the apparent inefficiency of immunity in man, the species specificity of immune responses and, until recently, the limited availability of parasite material. Immunization using dead or irradiated parasites has been achieved successfully in a variety of experimental model systems and, although similar vaccines are not likely to be suitable for use in man, they have illuminated some of the approaches that are likely to be fruitful. Indeed, research that has developed from these approaches has renewed optimism that vaccines effective in man can be produced.

There are currently three targets for vaccination against malaria, the sporozoite, the merozoite and the gametocytes. Most emphasis is placed upon the first two, control of which would directly benefit the recipient of the vaccine. In both cases, as was discussed in Chapter 3, the advent of monoclonal antibodies has allowed a much more precise knowledge of antigens which are important for the normal development of the infection. A number of protective antigens have been identified in the merozoite and schizont stages of both experimental models (*P. yoelii* in mice, *P. knowlesi* in primates) and human malarias (*P. falciparum*). In the latter, four schizont-specific antigens have been characterized and shown to be targets for antibody in *in vitro* tests of immunity. Three of these antigens, with molecular weights of 200 kD, 140 kD and 82 kD are also known to be recognized by antibodies present in sera of patients from areas in which *falciparum* malaria is endemic and may therefore represent major protective antigens. Use of such antigens in a potential vaccine requires their availability in far larger amounts than is possible using *in vitro* culture techniques and production using DNA-recombinant technology is being actively pursued. Much greater progress has been made with the protective surface antigens of the sporozoite stage. Using appropriate monoclonals, surface antigens have been identified and characterized in several species, including *P. falciparum*. Compared with the protective antigens of the merozoite stage those of the sporozoite are smaller (Table 10.2). Surface labelling shows that the antigen covers the entire sporozoite surface and that this protein is derived from high molecular weight, intracellular precursors. Binding and inhibition studies have established that the number of antigenic determinants available on the surface protein is limited and this has facilitated the use of *in vitro* translation and of cloning procedures. Using total RNA extracted from the thoraxes of control and *P. knowlesi*-infected mosquitoes, it has been possible to prepare double-stranded cDNA, insert into plasmids and clone in *E. coli*. Recombinant organisms could be screened easily for the sporozoite antigen

Table 10.2 Sporozoite antigens of *Plasmodium* species. Molecular weights of surface antigen protein and internal precursors. (Data from Turner, 1983, *Immunology Today*, **4**, 123.)

Species	Mol. weight of surface antigen (kD)	Mol. weight of precursors (kD)
P. berghei	44	52, 54
P. cynomolgi	48	56, 58
P. falciparum	58	65, 67
P. knowlesi	42	50, 52

using specific monoclonals and successful recombinants have been isolated. Production of the antigen in this way has allowed detailed sequence analysis and the identification of a dodecapeptide sequence which reacts with anti-sporozoite monoclonal antibody. The way is now open to test this peptide as a vaccine in the *P. knowlesi* system and, if successful, to apply a similar approach to the human malarias.

Although sporozoite vaccination is known to confer immunity (see Chapter 3) it is unlikely that vaccination with biosynthetically produced sporozoite antigen can ever be the sole form of protection against malaria. The stage specificity of malarial immunity means that immunity against sporozoite stages will not protect against erythrocytic stages. Thus unless vaccination is 100% effective, and of course that can never be guaranteed, some sporozoites will become established and disease will follow. It is therefore necessary to develop an anti-merozoite vaccine, which will protect against the pathogenic stage of infection, and the demonstration that it is possible to clone genes coding for protective antigens of the sporozoite has given this work an important impetus.

10.5.2   Schistosomiasis

The basic parameters for vaccination strategies have been laid down by laboratory studies which have clearly identified the early larval stages of infection as being both immunogenic and susceptible to immunologically-mediated attack. Stimulation of immunity with antigens extracted from parasite stages has in general been totally ineffective, but many workers have shown that it is possible to vaccinate experimental animals using irradiation-attenuated cercariae or schistosomula. These organisms fail to mature in the host, thereby avoiding the pathological adult stage, but nevertheless stimulate high levels of immunity to challenge with normal larvae. The original laboratory experiments with irradiated vaccines were carried out in primates and rodents, but the logistic problems inherent in obtaining and storing quantities of larvae prevented extension of the work into large-scale field trials against schistosome infections in cattle and sheep. The development of successful techniques of cryopreservation solved this logistic problem and field trials against infections with *S. bovis* in cattle have been carried out in the Sudan. The trials used larvae that had been irradiated at 3 krad and were very successful in preventing many of the pathological consequences of infection (Fig. 10.5), although they were not completely successful in conferring total resistance to the establishment of adult worms and vaccinated animals continued to pass eggs. In the context of a vaccine for veterinary use this factor is not a major significance compared with the very marked increase in economic productivity seen in vaccinated animals compared with untreated controls. Clearly, however, this level of partial resistance is unlikely to be acceptable when a human vaccine is contemplated. Rather better results have been used in trials in primates using larvae irradiated at very high levels, 25 krad or more, at which level not only is good immunity stimulated, but the larvae die at an early stage, in the skin, and there is minimal risk of pathology.

Even with such improved results, it is unlikely that irradiation-attenuated organisms will ever be the basis for a completely safe and successful human vaccine. This is much more likely to come from the isolation and synthesis of a protective tegumental antigen, a field in which some success has already been achieved (see Chapter 5). Monoclonal antibodies which recognize tegumental antigens present on schistosomula of *S. mansoni* have been prepared and these antibodies can confer immunity *in vivo*. They have also been used to isolate and identify candidate antigens from tegumental fractions, and there is evidence that these antigens are recognized by antibodies in the sera of immune patients. *In vitro* translation of mRNA from

154

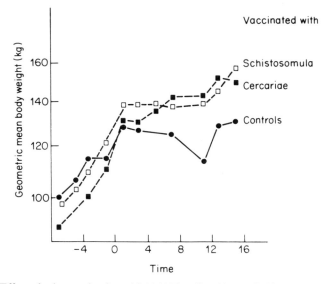

Fig. 10.5 Effect of prior vaccination with 10 000 irradiated larvae (schistosomula or cercaria) on growth of calves infected with 10 000 normal cercariae of *Schistosoma bovis*. Irradiated larvae were given week-8 and the challenge given on week 0. Schistosomula were given by intramuscular injection, cercariae percutaneously. At the end of the experiment the vaccinated calves had 43–50% fewer adult worms and 63–66% fewer eggs in their tissues than controls. (Data from Bushara *et al.*, 1978, *Parasitology*, **77**, 303.)

S. mansoni has also been achieved, as has a limited degree of gene cloning. All of these factors are hopeful pointers to the possibility of devising an effective vaccine along the lines discussed in section 10.4.3.

Although vaccination against infection is the most important strategy that is envisaged for the immunologically-based control of schistosomiasis, it is not the only one. Another is vaccination to prevent or minimize the pathological consequences of infection, a rather more controversial approach. Schistosomiasis is, *par excellence*, an infection that produces disease of immunopathological origin. As already discussed in Chapter 5, the pathological consequences of infection arise primarily from DTH responses directed against antigens released from the eggs. These antigens have now been characterized in great detail. There is good *in vivo* evidence, from laboratory and clinical studies, that the degree of responsiveness to egg antigen is modulated as infection progresses, and *in vitro* studies have implicated both antibody and suppressor cell activity in this modulation. It should therefore be possible to think in terms of using purified or synthesized egg antigens to induce regulatory responses and thus decrease the degree of pathology (granuloma size) without losing the protective value of the local antigen sequestration that appears to be associated with granuloma formation in *S. mansoni* at least. Without this sequestion there is focal necrosis of liver tissue, a pathological condition that is more severe than granuloma formation. However, even if practicable, it remains to be seen whether such an approach to vaccination will ever be considered ethical, since infection as such will not be controlled.

References and Further Reading

Journals

Original papers on immunoparasitology appear in a wide range of journals. Some of the major journals are listed below.

Acta Tropica
Advances in Parasitology
American Journal of Tropical Medicine and Hygiene
Australian Journal of Experimental Biology and Medical Science
Bulletin of the World Health Organization
Clinical and Experimental Immunology
Experimental Parasitology
Immunology
Infection and Immunity
International Journal for Parasitology
Journal of Immunology
Journal of Infectious Diseases
Journal of Parasitology
Parasite Immunology
Parasitology
Research in Veterinary Science
Transactions of the Royal Society of Tropical Medicine and Hygiene
Tropenmedizin and Parasitologie
Veterinary Parasitology

Textbooks and reviews

The references listed below are intended to amplify the chapters in the present book and to provide an introduction to the wider literature in each field. Original research papers have not been included (with a few exceptions) as these can be obtained from the bibliographies of the works cited.

References

Chapter One

Chandler, A.C. & Read, C.P. (1961). *Introduction to Parasitology*. John Wiley, London.
Cox, F.E.G. (editor) (1982). *Modern Parasitology*. Blackwell Scientific Publications, Oxford.
Donaldson, R.J. (editor) (1979). *Parasites and Western Man*. M.T.P. Press, Lancaster.
Kennedy, C.R. (editor) (1976). *Ecological Aspects of Parasitology*. North-Holland, Amsterdam.
Keusch, G.T. (editor) (1982). The Biology of Parasitic Infection. *Reviews of Infectious Diseases.*, **4**, 735–911.
Kreier, J.P. (197–8). *Parasitic Protozoa*, Vols. 1–3. Academic Press, New York.
Knight, R. (1982). *Parasitic Disease in Man*. Churchill Livingstone, Edinburgh.
Mims, C.A. (1982). *The Pathogenesis of Infectious Disease*. Academic Press, New York.
Muller, R. (1975). *Worms and Disease. A Manual of Medical Helminthology*. Heinemann Medical Books Ltd, London.
Peters, W. & Giles, H.M. (1977). *Colour Atlas of Tropical Medicine and Parasitology*. Wolfe Medical Publications, London.
Smyth, J.D. (1976). *Introduction to Animal Parasitology*. Hodder & Stoughton, London.
Soulsby, E.J.L. (1982). *Helminths, Arthropods and Protozoa of Domesticated Animals*. Balliere & Tindall, London.
Whitfield, P.S. (1979). *The Biology of Parasitism*. Edward Arnold, London.

Chapter Two

(1) General Texts
Fudenberg, H.H. *et al.* (editors) (1978). *Basic and Clinical Immunology*. Lange Medical Publications, California.
Golub, E.S. (1981). *The Cellular Basis of the Immune Response*. Sinauer Associates, Inc., Massachusetts.
Klein, J. (1982). *Immunology _ The Science of Self-Non-Self Discrimination*. John Wiley, New York.
McConnel, I., Munro, A. & Waldman, H. (1981). *The Immune System: a Course on the Molecular and Cellular Basis of Immunity*. Blackwell Scientific Publications, Oxford.
Roitt, I. (1980). *Essential Immunology*. Blackwell Scientific Publications, Oxford.

(2) Effector Mechanisms
Askenase, P.W. (1977). Role of basophils, mast cells and vasoamines in hypersensitivity reactions with a delayed time course. *Progress in Allergy*, **23**, 199.
Butterworth, A.E., Vadas, M.A. & David, J.R. (1980). Mechanisms of eosinophil-mediated helminthotoxicity. In: *The Eosinophil in Health and Disease*, p. 253 (ed. A.A.F. Mahmound & K.F. Austen). Grune & Stratton, New York.
Capron, A. *et al.* (1982). Antibody-dependent cell-mediated cytotoxicity against parasites. *Progress in Allergy*, **31**, 234.
Colley, D.G. & James, S.L. (1979). Participation of eosinophils in immunological systems. In: *Cellular, Molecular and Clinical Aspects of Allergic Disorders: Comprehensive Immunology*, Vol. 6, p. 55 (ed. S. Gupta & R.A. Good). Plenum Press, New York.

Dessaint, J.P. (1982). Anaphylactic antibodies and their significance (in Capron, 1982, p. 621).
Elliner, J.J. & Mahmoud, A.A.F. (1982). Phagocytes and worms: David and Goliath revisited. *Reviews of Infectious Diseases.*, **4**, 698.
Jarrett, E.E.E. & Miller, H.R.P. (1982). Production and activities of IgE in helminth infection. *Progress in Allergy*, **31**, 178.
Joseph, M. (1982). Effector functions of phagocyte cells against the helminths (in Capron, 1982, p. 567).
Leid, W.R. & Williams, J.F. (1979). Helminth parasites and the host inflammatory system. In: *Chemical Zoology*, Vol. 11, p. 229 (eds. M. Florkin & B. Scheer). Academic Press, New York.
Santoro, F. (1982). Interaction of complement with parasite surfaces (in Capron, 1982, p. 639).
Willmott, S. (editor) (1980). *The Eosinophil in Tropical Disease. Transactions of the Royal Society for Tropical Medicine and Hygiene.*, **74**, (Suppl.), 1–63.
Willmott, S. (editor) (1983). *Symposium on the Macrophage. Transactions of the Royal Society for Tropical Medicine and Hygiene*, **77**, 597.

Chapter Three

Anders, R.F. *et al.* (1982). Parasite antigens and methods of analysis (in Cohen & Warren, 1982, p. 28).
Barriga, O.O. (1981). *The Immunology of Parasitic Infections.* M.T.P. Press, Lancaster.
Bloom, B.R. (1979). Games parasites play: how parasites evade immune surveillance. *Nature*, **279**, 21.
Van Den Bossche, H. (editor) (1980). *The Host-Invader Interplay.* Elsevier/North-Holland Biochemical Press, Amsterdam.
Capron, A. (1982). Immunoparasitology. *Clinics in Immunology and Allergy*, **2**, 487.
Ciba Foundation Symposium No. 25. (1974). *Parasites in the Immunized Host: Mechanisms of Survival.* Elsevier/North-Holland, Amsterdam.
Cohen, S. & Warren, K.S. (1982). *Immunology of Parasitic Infections.* Blackwell Scientific Publications, Oxford.
Davies, A.J.S. *et al.* (1980). The biological significance of the immune response with special reference to parasites and cancer. *Journal of Parasitology*, **66**, 705.
Frank, W. (editor) (1982). *Immune Reactions to Parasites.* Gustav Fischer Verlag, Stuttgart.
Mansfield, J.M. (editor) (1981). *Parasitic Diseases*, Vol. 1. *The Immunology.* Marcel Dekker, Inc., New York and Basel.
Mauel, J. (1982). Effector and escape mechanisms in host-parasite relationships. *Progress in Allergy*, **31**, 1.
Mitchell, G.F. (1979). Effector cells, molecules and mechanisms in host-protective immunity to parasites. *Immunology*, **38**, 209.
Mitchell, G.F. (1980). Responses to infection with metazoan and protozoan parasites in mice. *Advances in Immunology*, **28**, 451.
Mitchell, G.F. & Anders, R.F. (1982). Parasite antigens and their immunogenicity in infected hosts. In: *The Antigens*, Vol. 6, p. 69 (ed. M. Sela). Academic Press, New York.
Owen, D.G. (editor) (1982). *Animal Models in Parasitology.* MacMillan, London.
Pery, P. & Luffau, G. (1979). Antigens of helminths. In: *The Antigens*, Vol. 5, p. 83 (ed. M. Sela). Academic Press, New York.
Playfair, J.H.L. (1978). Effective and ineffective responses to parasites: evidence from experimental models. *Current Topics in Microbiology and Immunology*, **80**, 37.
Sprent, J.F.A. (1969), Evolutionary aspects of immunity in zooparasitic infections. In: *Immunity to Parasitic Animals*, Vol. 1, p. 3. (eds. G.J. Jackson, R. Herman & I. Singer). North-Holland, Amsterdam.

Chapter Four

(1) Malaria

Brown, K.N. (1982). Host Resistance to Malaria. *Critical Reviews in Tropical Medicine*, **1**, (ed. R.K. Chandra). Plenum Press, New York.
Cohen, S. (1979). Immunity to malaria. *Proceedings of the Royal Society of London* (B), **203**, 323.

Cohen, S. & Lambert, P.H. (1982). Malaria (in Cohen & Warren, 1982, p. 422).
Cohen, S. *et al.* (1961). Gamma globulin and acquired immunity to human malaria. *Nature*, **192**, 733.
Cox, F.E.G. (1982). Non-specific immunity against parasites (in Capron, 1982, p. 705).
Jayawardena, A.N. (1981). Immune responses in malaria (in Mansfield, 1981, p. 85).
Killick-Kendrick, R. & Peters, W. (editors) (1978). *Rodent Malaria*. Academic Press, New York.
Nussenzweig, R.S. *et al.* (1978). Immunological responses (in Killick-Kendrick & Peters, 1978, p. 247).
World Health Organization (1979). Immunology of Malaria. *Bulletin of the World Health Organization*, **57**, 1–290.
World Health Organization (1979). *Role of the Spleen in the Immunology of Parasitic Diseases*. Tropical Diseases Research Series 1. Schwabe & Co. AG, Basel.
Yoshida, N. *et al.* (1980). Hybridoma produces protective antibodies directed against the sporozoite stage of malaria parasite. *Science*, **207**, 71.

(2)   Leishmania
Blackwell, J.M. (1982). Genetic control of recovery from visceral leishmaniasis. *Transactions of the Royal Society of Tropical Medicine and Hygiene*, **76**, 147.
Bradley, D.J. (1980). Genetic control of resistance to protozoal infections. In: *Genetic Control of Natural Resistance to Infections and Malignancy*, p. 9 (eds. E. Skamene, P. Kongshavn & M. Landy). Academic Press, New York.
Howard, J.G. *et al.* (1982). Genetically determined response mechanisms to cutaneous leishmaniasis. *Transaction of the Royal Society of Tropical Medicine and Hygiene*, **76**, 152.
Killick-Kendrick, R. & Peters, W. (editors) (1983). *Leishmaniasis*. Academic Press, New York.
Mavel, J. & Behin, R. (1982). Leishmaniasis (in Cohen & Warren, 1982, p. 299).
Reed, S.G. (1981). Immunology of *Leishmania* infections (in Mansfield, 1981, p. 291).

Chapter Five

Cross, G.A.M. (1978). Antigenic variation in trypanosomes. *Proceedings of the Royal Society London B*, **202**, 55.
Diggs, C.L. (1982). Immunological research on African trypanosomiasis. *Progress in Allergy*, **31**, 268.
Hoeijmakers, J.H.J. *et al.* (1980). Novel expression-linked copies of the genes for variant surface antigens in trypanosomes. *Nature*, **284**, 78.
Mansfield, J.M. (1981). Immunology and immunopathology of African trypanosomiasis (in Mansfield, 1981, p. 167).
Murray, M. *et al.* (1982). Host susceptibility to African trypanosomiasis: trypanotolerance. *Advances in Parasitology*, **21**, 2.
Turner, M.J. (1982). Biochemistry of the variant surface glycoproteins of salivarian trypanosomes. *Advances in Parasitology*, **21**, 70.
Vickerman, K. (1978). Antigenic variation in trypanosomes. *Nature*, **273**, 613.
Vickerman, K. & Barry, J.D. (1982). African trypanosomiasis (in Cohen & Warren, 1982, p. 204).

Chapter Six

Butterworth, A.E. *et al.* (1982). Studies on the mechanisms of immunity in human schistosomiasis. *Immunological Reviews*, **61**, 5.
Capron, A. *et al.* (1982). Effector mechanisms of immunity to schistosomes and their regulation. *Immunological Reviews*, **61**, 41.
Clegg, J.A. (1974). Host antigens and the immune response in schistosomiasis (in CIBA Symposium, 1974, p. 161).
Colley, D.G. (1981). Immune responses and immunoregulation in experimental and clinical schistosomiasis (in Mansfield, 1981, p. 1).
McLaren, D.J. (1980). *Schistosoma mansoni: The Parasite Surface in Relation to Host Immunity*. John Wiley & Sons, Chichester, England.

Phillips, S.M. & Colley, D.G. (1978). Immunological aspects of host responses to schistosomiasis: resistance, immunopathology and eosinophil involvement. *Progress in Allergy*, **24**, 49.
Smithers, S.R. & Doenhoff, M.J. (1982). Schistosomiasis (in Cohen & Warren, 1982, p. 527).
Warren, K.S. (1972). The immunopathogenesis of schistosomiasis: a multidisciplinary approach. *Transactions of the Royal Society of Tropical Medicine and Hygiene*, **66**, 417.
Warren, K.S. (1977). Modulation of immunopathology and disease in schistosomiasis. *American Journal of Tropical Medicine and Hygiene*, **26** (Suppl.), 113.
Warren, K.S. (1978). Regulation of the prevalence and intensity of schistosomiasis in man. Immunology or ecology? *Journal of Infectious Diseases*, **127**, 595.

Chapter Seven

Befus, A.D. & Bienenstock, J. (1982). Factors involved in symbiosis and host-resistance at the mucosa-parasite interface. *Progress in Allergy*, **31**, 76.
Bienenstock, J. & Befus, A.D. (1980). Review. Mucosal immunology. *Immunology*, **41**, 249.
Catty, D. & Ross, I.N. (1979). Immunological aspects of infection with gastrointestinal parasites (protozoa and nematodes). In: *Immunity of the Gastrointestinal Tract*, p. 246 (ed. P. Asquith). Churchill Livingstone, Edinburgh.
Marsden, P.D.L. (editor) (1978). Intestinal Parasites. *Clinics in Gastroenterology*, **7**, 1–243.
Miller, H.R.P. (1980). The structure, origin and function of mucosal mast cells. A brief review. *Biologie Cellulaire*, **39**, 229.
Ogilvie, B.M. & Love, R.J. (1974). Cooperation between antibodies and cells in immunity to a nematode parasite. *Transplantation Review*, **19**, 147.
Ogilvie, B.M. & Parrott, D.V.M. (1977). The immunological consequences of nematode infection. In: *Immunology of the Gut*, CIBA Foundation Symposium 46, p. 183. Elsevier, Amsterdam.
Soulsby, E.J.L. (1979). The immune system and helminth infection in domestic species. *Advances in Veterinary Science and Comparative Medicine*, **23**, 71.
Wakelin, D. (1978). Immunity to intestinal parasites. *Nature*, **273**, 617.
Wakelin, D. & Denham, D.A. (1983). The immune response. In: *Trichinella and Trichinosis*, p. 265 (ed. W.C. Campbell). Plenum Press, New York.

Chapter Eight

Denham, D.A. & McGreevy, P.B. (1977). Brugian filariasis: epidemiological and experimental studies. *Advances in Parasitology*, **15**, 243.
Mackenzie, C.D. (1983). *Host Response and Clinical Disease in Onchocerciasis*. John Wiley & Sons, Chichester, England.
Maizels, R.M. *et al.* (1982). Molecules on the surface of parasitic nematodes as probes of the immune response in infection. *Immunological Review*, **61**, 109.
Nelson, G.S. (1970). Onchocerciasis. *Advances in Parasitology*, **8**, 173.
Ogilvie, B.M. & Mackenzie, C.D. (1981). Immunology and immunopathology of infection caused by filarial nematodes (in Mansfield, 1981, p. 227).
Piessens, W.F. & Mackenzie, C.D. (1982). Immunology of lymphatic filariasis and onchocerciasis (in Cohen & Warren, 1982, p. 622).

Chapter Nine

Askenase, P.W. (1979). Immunopathology of parasitic diseases: involvement of basophils and mast cells. *Springer Seminars in Immunopathology*, **4**, 1.
Benjamini, E. & Feingold, B.F. (1970). Immunity to arthropods. In: *Immunity to Parasitic Animals*, Vol. 2, p. 1016 (eds. G.J. Jackson, R. Herman & I. Singer). Appleton-Century-Crofts, New York.
Brown, S.J. & Askenase, P.W. (1983). Immune rejection of ectoparasites (ticks) by T cell and IgG$_1$ antibody recruitment of basophils and eosinophils. *Federation Proceedings*, **42**, 1744.
Wikel, S.K. (1980). Host resistance to tick-borne pathogens by virtue of resistance to tick infestation. *Annals of Tropical Medicine and Parasitology*, **74**, 103.
Willadsen, P. (1980). Immunity to ticks. *Advances in Parasitology*, **18**, 293.

Chapter Ten

Chedid, L. (1977). Therapeutic potential of immunoregulating synthetic compounds. In: *Immunity in Parasitic Diseases*, p. 249. Colloque INSERM 72. INSERM, Paris.

Clegg, J. & Smith, M.A. (1978). Prospects for the development of dead vacines against helminths. *Advances in Parasitology*, **16**, 165.

Cohen, S. & Mitchell, G.H. (1978). Prospects for immunization against malaria. *Current Topics in Microbiology and Immunology.*, **80**, 97.

Cox, F.E.G. (1978). Specific and nonspecific immunization against parasitic infections. *Nature*, **273**, 623.

Cross, G.A.M. (1982). New technologies for parasitology. In: *Parasites: Their World and Ours*, p. 3 (eds. D.F. Mettrick & S.S. Desser). Elsevier Biomedical Press. Amsterdam.

Hommel, M. (1981). Malaria: immunity and prospects for vaccination. *Western Journal of Medicine*, **135**, 285.

Houba, V. & Chan, S.H. (editors) (1982). *Properties of the Monoclonal Antibodies Produced by Hybridoma Technology and their Application to the Study of Diseases*. UNDP/World Bank/WHO Special Programme for Research and Training in Tropical Diseases, Geneva.

Lloyd, S. (1981). Progress in immunization against parasitic helminths. *Parasitology*, **83**, 225.

Miller, T.A. (1978). Industrial development and field use of the canine hookworm vaccine. *Advances in Parasitology*, **16**, 333.

Mitchell, G.F. (1982). New trends towards vaccination against parasties (in Capron, 1982, p. 721).

Rowe, D.S. (1977). Vaccines and other immunological approaches to the control of parasitic diseases: needs and prospects. In: *Immunity in Parasitic Diseases*, p. 307. Colloque INSERM, 72. INSERM, Paris.

Smithers, S.R. (1980). Vaccination against schistosomiasis. In: *New Developments with Human and Veterinary Vaccines*, p. 287. Alan R. Liss Inc., New York.

Taylor, A.E.R. & Muller, R. (editors) (1980). *Vaccination against Parasites*, Symposia of the British Society for Parasitology, Vol. 18. Blackwell Scientific Publications, Oxford.

Urquhart, G.M. (1980). Application of immunity in the control of parasitic disease. *Veterinary Parasitology*, **6**, 217.

Wakelin, D. (1983). Immunity to helminths and prospects for control. *Critical Reviews of Tropical Medicine*, **2**, (in press).

Index

Bold type indicates pages with illustrations or tables.